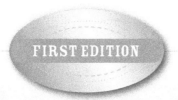

FIRST EDITION

D1086409

COGNITIVE REHABILITATION MANUAL

TRANSLATING EVIDENCE-BASED RECOMMENDATIONS INTO PRACTICE

Primary Author   **Edmund C. Haskins, PhD**
Hook Rehabilitation Center, Indianapolis, Indiana

Contributing Authors and Editors

Keith Cicerone, PhD, ABPP-Cn, FACRM
JFK Johnson Rehabilitation Institute, Edison, New Jersey

Kristen Dams-O'Connor, PhD
Mount Sinai School of Medicine, New York, New York

Rebecca Eberle, MA, CCC-SLP
Indiana University, Bloomington, Indiana

Donna Langenbahn, PhD, FACRM
Rusk Institute of Rehabilitation Medicine, New York, New York

Amy Shapiro-Rosenbaum, PhD
Park Terrace Care Center, Flushing, New York

Managing Editor   **Lance E. Trexler, PhD**
Rehabilitation Hospital of Indiana, Indianapolis, Indiana

WITHDRAWN
TOURO COLLEGE LIBRARY

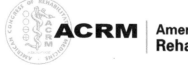

ACRM | **American Congress of Rehabilitation Medicine**

Brain Injury-Interdisciplinary Special Interest Group (BI-ISIG)

KH

126

Produced by ACRM Publishing

ACRM | American Congress of Rehabilitation Medicine

SINCE 1923

GLOBAL MULTIDISCIPLINARY REHABILITATION RESEARCH

www.ACRM.org

ACRM Leadership

President Tamara Bushnik, PhD, FACRM
Chief Executive Officer Jon W. Lindberg, MBA, CAE

ISBN: 978-0615538877   EDFICS0204

ACRM HEADQUARTERS
11654 Plaza America Drive, Suite 535
Reston, Virginia, USA 20190
Tel: +1.317.471.8760
Fax: +1.866.692.1619
Email: info@ACRM.org

9/29/20

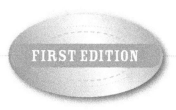

"A concise and precise manual that is excellent for therapists, professors and students in the field of cognitive rehabilitation."

ADA LEUNG, PhD
UNIVERSITY OF ALBERTA, EDMONTON, AB (CAN)

"Bible for new and intermediate cognitive rehabilitation therapists."

JESSICA MARTINEZ, OTR
SCRIPPS, ENCINITAS, CA (USA)

"This Manual was just what I was looking for. It provides me with a step-by-step approach to provide quality treatments. The decision trees keep me focused and on the right path."

MERRI VITSE, COTA/L
MAYO CLINIC, ROCHESTER, MN (USA)

"This is a must-have publication if you are currently practicing or plan to practice in the area of cognitive rehabilitation."

STEPHANIE RITTER OTR/L
MAYO CLINIC, ROCHESTER, MN (USA)

"Useful for both experienced professionals in cognitive rehabilitation and for a first approach."

PAOLO BOLDRINI, MD
OSPEDALE CA' FONCELLO, PIAZZALE OSPEDALE
TREVISO (ITA)

"The Cognitive Rehabilitation Manual is a comprehensive collection of evidence-based research practices organized in a clear manner. The information is presented in a format that will benefit both seasoned professionals and entry level clinicians working with patients who present with cognitive/communication deficits."

DAVID J. HAJJAR, MS, CCC-SLP
CROTCHED MOUNTAIN FOUNDATION, GREENFIELD, NH
(USA)

"This manual has moved the post-acute brain injury industry significantly forward by providing clear guidelines for delivering 'best practice' cognitive rehabilitation."

SID DICKSON, PhD, ABPP
PATE REHABILITATION, DALLAS, TX (USA)

"The CRM has the potential to unite allied health practitioners, and revolutionize the way in which they provide comprehensive, holistic cognitive rehabilitation to survivors of acquired brain injury."

MICHAEL FRAAS, PhD
OAK PARK, IL (USA)

"The manual is well aimed at ACBIS qualified staff and clinical psychologists and occupational therapists. It covers many of the well-researched and presented single or small-n case studies and the larger group outcome studies up to the present. It is certainly evidence-based in my view and it succeeds in translating the disparate evidence base in the clinical literature to workable recommendations for staff on the ground."

DR BRIAN WALDRON
ACQUIRED BRAIN INJURY, DUBLIN (IRL)

"Dr. Haskins and his team provided a very in-depth and precise perspective to cognitive remediation therapy and the goals and objectives needed to meet these needs."

JEFFREY A. FALLERONI, MSCCC/SLP
REMED, PITTSBURGH, PA (USA)

"Cognitive rehabilitation is a dynamic practice between the clinician and the client, not fitting into a typical treatment protocol. This manual provides the kind of support that clinicians need to develop effective and evidence-based treatment plans."

JESSICA PETERSEN, OTR/L
MAYO CLINIC, ROCHESTER, MN (USA)

"The Cognitive Rehabilitation Manual is a landmark volume translating decades of research into clearly described procedures indispensable for working clinicians. This manual is an invaluable guide to the evidence-based practice of cognitive rehabilitation for clinicians with or without strong research backgrounds."

JAMES F. MALEC, PhD, ABPP-CN, RP, FACRM
REHABILITATION HOSPITAL OF INDIANA, INDIANAPOLIS,
IN (USA)

"Thoughtfully organized, practical, and invaluable — this manual provides step-by-step techniques for delivering cognitive therapies. This promises to be an essential guide to the delivery of cognitive rehabilitation services for persons with brain injury."

RONALD T. SEEL, PhD
SHEPHERD CENTER, ATLANTA, GA (USA)

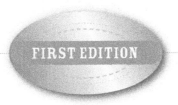

"The *Cognitive Rehabilitation Manual; Translating Evidence-Based Recommendations into Practice* is a guide for clinicians who want to effectively deliver evidence-based rehabilitation interventions in everyday clinical practice. The Brain Injury Interdisciplinary Special Interest Group (BI-ISIG) of the American Congress of Rehabilitation Medicine (ACRM) is committed to fostering the use of empirically supported interventions to improve the lives of individuals with brain injury. A series of reviews, which are published in the *Archives of Physical Medicine and Rehabilitation* (Cicerone et al., 2000; 2005; 2011) have reviewed the scientific literature and put forth standards and guidelines for clinical practice based on the quality of evidence available for each intervention. The *Cognitive Rehabilitation Manual* operationalizes or "translates" these guidelines into step-by-step procedures that can be used by clinicians who treat individuals with brain injury.

The volume is organized into six chapters. The introductory chapter compiles the clinical wisdom of the authors into a practical roadmap for structuring and implementing cognitive rehabilitation interventions. Treatment considerations and patient factors that may influence the course of treatment are discussed, and a guide to goal-setting that is applied throughout the manual is introduced. Subsequent chapters present practical guides for the implementation of evidence-based interventions for impairments in each of the following areas: Executive Functions, Memory, Attention, Hemispatial Neglect, and Social Communication. The content of each chapter draws from empirically-supported rehabilitation interventions included in the Cicerone et al. reviews (2000; 2005; 2011) and the collective clinical experience of the authors of the *Cognitive Rehabilitation Manual.*

Wherever possible, step-by-step guidelines for implementing each intervention and setting relevant individual goals are provided, along with clinical recommendations for tailoring and modifying the intervention according to patients' needs. In cases where in-depth treatment manuals exist, full references and links to these materials are provided. Additional appendices include rubrics for goal-setting in each of these domains of functioning, and handouts or worksheets that can be used to record and evaluate progress.

The *Manual* is ideally suited for clinicians who have had some formal training in cognitive rehabilitation and who have experience working with individuals with brain injury (e.g., traumatic brain injury, stroke). The interventions described can be readily used by occupational therapists, speech and language therapists, psychologists, and other rehabilitation professionals.

The *Cognitive Rehabilitation Manual; Translating Evidence-Based Recommendations into Practice* is a significant contribution to the field of brain injury rehabilitation. Never before have research outcomes been made so accessible for use in everyday clinical work. This important volume will raise the bar in cognitive rehabilitation by aiding clinicians in delivering high-quality, empirically-supported interventions to improve the lives of the patients we serve.

KRISTEN DAMS-O'CONNOR, PhD
MOUNT SINAI SCHOOL OF MEDICINE, NEW YORK, NY (USA)

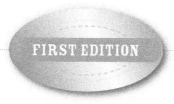

FIRST EDITION

Acknowledgements

The ACRM BI-ISIG Cognitive Rehabilitation Task Force Manual Committee acknowledges the following individuals for their review and comment on this manual:

Teresa Ashman, PhD, Samantha Backhaus, PhD, Julie Balzano, MA, Tom Bergquist, PhD, Elisabeth Bond, PhD, Cynthia Braden, PhD, Catherine Breen, MA, Joshua Cantor, PhD, Christine Dorantes, BA, Michael Fraas, PhD, Yelena Goldin-Loretta, PhD, Nora Goudsmit, PhD, J. Preston Harley, PhD, Chari Hirshson, PhD, Nicole Holzworth, BS, Jason Krellman, PhD, Linda Laatsch, PhD, Jim Malec, PhD, Yuka Matsuzawa, PsyD, Gina Mitchell, MA, Susan Paradise, MEd, Jeff Snell, PhD, and Jack Thomas, MS.

Preface

This manual was developed by a sub-group of the Cognitive Rehabilitation Task Force of the Brain Injury Interdisciplinary Special Interest Group (BI-ISIG) of the American Congress of Rehabilitation Medicine (ACRM). It is modeled on a manual that was developed by Edmund Haskins, Ph.D., at Hook Rehabilitation Center in the Community Health Network in Indianapolis, Indiana. The current manual reflects the evidence-based treatment recommendations put forth by the BI-ISIG Cognitive Rehabilitation Task Force of ACRM and the clinical experience and expertise of the authors as discussed in the Introduction (see Section 1.1).

Dedication

Cognitive rehabilitation is by some standards a relatively new field. Anyone who has worked with a person with brain injury and their family is aware of the importance of cognitive recovery to them. While the humanitarian recognition of the need to promote recovery of cognitive functions following brain injury is not new, the scientific basis for cognitive rehabilitation is.

Nonetheless, while the history of science in cognitive rehabilitation may be recent, the number and sophistication of empirical studies have accelerated remarkably over the last 30 years such that we now have the scientific evidence to guide clinical practice. Without the contributions of Leonard Diller, PhD and Keith Cicerone, PhD, we would not be at this historical intersection.

Lance E. Trexler, PhD
Donna Langenbahn, PhD
J. Preston Harley, PhD
July 19, 2011

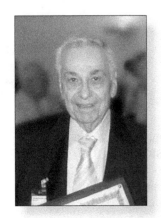

Leonard Diller, PhD having started at the [Rusk] Institute of Rehabilitation Medicine at NYU Medical Center in 1952, is now approaching his 60th year in rehabilitation. He assumed a leadership role at Rusk as the new field of medical rehabilitation sought to assess and meet the clinical and functional needs of individuals with disability, to train clinicians and researchers, and to gain a foothold in cultural and political arenas. In this context, Dr. Diller built a psychology program where clinical observation, beginning with the patient, fueled intervention protocols and research, and the research, in turn, sought to validate obtained results. His approach to the problem of brain injury treatment and research was direct and elegant, backed by scientific logic: develop a standard task sensitive to the problem, elucidate behavior by examining task response style, determine task conditions that increase or decrease the problem, and develop a methodology to increase awareness and enable the individual to overcome the problem while performing a skilled activity. In sum, he taught us that neuropsychological knowledge and process could help us design and guide rehabilitation procedures. This methodology formed the basis for an astoundingly prolific research output, much of it seminal research in the area of acquired brain injury, and caused him to be regarded as "the founder of scientifically-based cognitive rehabilitation."[1] Innumerable individuals with brain injury, family members, clinicians, and researchers have benefited from Dr. Diller's gifts, and those who know him are awed by his enduring encyclopedic knowledge, kindness, and humility.

Innumerable individuals with brain injury, family members, clinicians, and researchers have benefited from Dr. Diller's gifts, and those who know him are awed by his enduring encyclopedic knowledge, kindness, and humility.

---

[1] Goldstein, G. (2009). Neuropsychology in New York City (1930-1960), *Archives of Clinical Neuropsychology, 24*, 137-143.

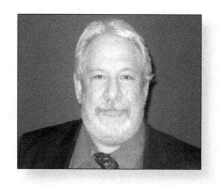

Keith Cicerone, PhD has been a clinician and researcher for over 30 years, and as such, has improved the quality of life for thousands of patients who have suffered brain injuries. It is clearly evident from his numerous publications and research that Dr. Cicerone had the wisdom to listen and learn from his patients. His concern for the well-being of individuals with brain injury has not been limited to clinical care. At the same time, he committed himself to improving the science behind his clinical practice. He has made significant contributions to the development of national policies recognizing cognitive rehabilitation as an effective treatment for individuals with brain injuries. In addition to conducting his own research, Dr. Cicerone led the American Congress of Rehabilitation Medicine, Brain Injury-Interdisciplinary Special Interest Group's evidence-based reviews, which were published in the *Archives of Physical Medicine and Rehabilitation* in 2000, 2005 and 2011. The present work is primarily based upon the findings and recommendations of these three publications. His leadership and commitment in the establishment of guidelines for cognitive rehabilitation have made it now possible to offer clinical practitioners of cognitive rehabilitation treatment strategies that are based upon scientific, empirical evidence.

COGNITIVE REHABILITATION MANUAL

TRANSLATING EVIDENCE-BASED RECOMMENDATIONS INTO PRACTICE

Table of Contents

CHAPTER 2
Rehabilitation For Impairments of Executive Functions

CHAPTER 3
Rehabilitation for Impairments of Memory

CHAPTER 4
Rehabilitation for Impairments of Attention

CHAPTER 5
Rehabilitation of Hemispatial Neglect

CHAPTER 6
Rehabilitation of Impairments of Social Communication

APPENDIX A
Strategic and Tactical Goal Writing

APPENDIX B
General/Non-Specific Forms

List of Tables, Figures and Clinical Forms

Chapter 4
Rehabilitation for Impairments of Attention

Chapter 5
Rehabilitation of Hemispatial Neglect

1. Introduction: Principles of Cognitive Rehabilitation

1.1 Functions and Structure of this Manual

This manual was developed to guide clinicians who conduct cognitive rehabilitation for individuals with acquired brain injury. The clinical protocols contained herein reflect the recommendations made by the Cognitive Rehabilitation Task Force of the Brain Injury Interdisciplinary Special Interest Group (BI-ISIG) of the American Congress of Rehabilitation Medicine (ACRM). These researchers have conducted several systematic reviews of the cognitive rehabilitation literature (see Cicerone et al., 2000, 2005, 2011) and have recommended treatment approaches and strategies that have sufficient empirical evidence of efficacy in ameliorating cognitive impairments following brain injury.

The treatment strategies recommended by the BI-ISIG Cognitive Rehabilitation Task Force have been graded based on the strength of empirical evidence to support their use. Specifically, the term "Practice Standard" is used to designate those strategies which have shown "substantive evidence" of effectiveness." These are offered with the strongest recommendation. The term "Practice Guideline" designates those that have shown "probable effectiveness," and these are given the next strongest recommendation. The term "Practice Option" designates those treatment strategies believed to have shown "possible effectiveness" but require further research evidence for stronger recommendation (Cicerone, Dahlberg, Malec et al., 2005).

The BI-ISIG recommendations contained herein are based on empirical evidence as well as clinical experience and judgment to create a manual that fosters the application of high-quality, evidence-based interventions. In this manual, we have taken the committee's recommendations and developed detailed protocols to instruct and guide clinicians in their implementation. Accordingly, the manual includes protocols for the treatment of the following areas: executive functioning, memory, attention and concentration, visual neglect, and social communication. Each protocol draws heavily from one or more studies that formed the basis of the BI-ISIG recommendations. In addition to presenting global strategies, each protocol includes a section describing suggested methods for implementing these strategies and guidelines for setting specific tactical goals.

As previously noted, the techniques, interventions, procedures or training strategies herein presented (except in one instance as noted) were all included in the Cicerone et al., 2000, 2005, 2011 reviews and the interventions in the systematic reviews were based on treatment for people with traumatic brain injury or stroke. While driven by research as cited, the Introduction reflects the professional consensus of the authors and editors. We also present in the Introduction stages of treatment (Acquisition, Application, and Adaptation) which were clearly used in the research of Sohlberg and Mateer (1987a), but these stages of training were not explicitly utilized in the treatment methodologies of other studies. These stages of treatment are included as useful guides to clinical application. Lastly, the Manual provides suggested methods for goal setting at the end of each chapter and in Appendix A. While the authors and editors felt that these were very useful clinically to practicing therapists, they were not part of the treatment methodologies of the studies in the Cicerone et al., 2000, 2005, or 2011 reviews.

The evidence for rehabilitation of disorders of executive functions, memory and attention includes specific protocols as well as more "complex" programs of treatment characterized by multiple steps, sequences, and highly organized protocols. The chapters on Executive Functions and Memory have a section on "Complex Evidence-Based Programs" and group treatment protocols are included in these sections as well. Throughout the current volume, when a proprietary treatment manual is available from the developers of a given approach (for example, Attention Process Training (APT) as developed by Sohlberg and Mateer (1987b), or Group Interactive Structured Treatment (GIST) as developed by Hawley et al. (2010), we provide a synopsis of this intervention, along with references to available treatment manuals. When an existing treatment manual is freely available in the public domain (for example, Problem-solving Training, Rath et al., 2003), we have provided worksheets and handouts, along with references to existing manuals.

1.2   Limitations of this Manual

This manual is intended to serve as a guide to help trained clinicians effectively employ empirically-supported treatments for individuals with brain injury. This manual is **not** intended to provide a substitute for specialized training and supervision in the application of the strategies and tactics described here. Therapists using this manual should have at least basic training in the principles and methods of cognitive rehabilitation, and prior experience in working with a brain-injured population. Examples of such professionals include occupational therapists, speech and language therapists, psychologists, or other rehabilitation professionals who have completed specialized training. It is not recommended that rehabilitation professionals implement treatments for significant emotional and behavioral disorders without the direct involvement of a professional specifically trained in the management and treatment of those issues (e.g., a psychologist).

It should be noted that it is not the intent of this manual to provide a comprehensive review on the nature of cognitive functions or impairments. A basic description of each domain of cognitive function is provided in the introduction of each chapter followed by an overview on the effects of brain injury on that domain of cognitive functioning. Abundant neuropsychological resources are available for the interested reader who wants more information on the nature of specific cognitive domains.

Finally, it should be noted that the current manual is not all-inclusive, in that it does not include protocols for the treatment of either aphasia or apraxia, although there are existing standards of treatment for these disorders.

1.3   How to Use This Manual

Prior to using this manual, one should first read this introduction thoroughly to become familiar with the over-arching goals and process of cognitive rehabilitation, the various types of treatment strategies and tactics employed, as well as general treatment planning and goal setting processes. Once the current chapter has been reviewed, users can skip directly to the section that addresses the specific deficits relevant to a particular patient (e.g., Rehabilitation for Impairments of Memory). However, regardless of the treatment domain of interest, the Introduction should be used in conjunction with that section to ensure the most effective treatment. In particular, it is recommended that the user refer back to this chapter as necessary to review the stages of treatment, to assist in the selection of appropriate treatment strategies, and to assist in developing individualized treatment plans and goals. Furthermore, at the end of each chapter, as well as in Appendix A, sample goals are provided to assist in developing appropriate treatment plans for each deficit domain. Additionally, Appendix B provides sample templates for tracking progress in rehabilitation.

1.4 Primary Goals of Cognitive Rehabilitation

The primary goal of cognitive rehabilitation is to ameliorate injury-related deficits in order to maximize safety, daily functioning, independence, and quality of life. Progress is achieved in a stepwise manner, with an emphasis on the following long term goals:

Problem orientation, awareness and goal setting: Assisting the patient in recognizing the specific problem(s) that require intervention, and collaborating with the patient to establish meaningful short- and long-term goals. Goal setting should be a collaborative process when possible and is often a major therapeutic priority, especially in the beginning to help engage the patient in the therapeutic process. Additionally, the patient needs to have the opportunity to become aware of the impairments which affect their long-term goals, but in context of an emotionally supportive and positive relationship. It is important at this stage to identify and share with the patient their strengths and resources to ameliorate the feelings of embarrassment and compromised self-worth that many people experience. Different types of unawareness are addressed later in this chapter and the rehabilitation of impairments of awareness are addressed in the chapter on Impairments of Executive Functions.

Compensation: Providing individuals with the necessary tools to help them function effectively despite persistent or chronic impairments is often the end goal of cognitive rehabilitation. When a person's usual ways of doing things are no longer possible due to injury-related deficits, new ways of achieving similar outcomes must be identified. For example, the use of a Memory Notebook or planner may result in fewer missed appointments, though the underlying memory impairment remains.

Internalization: This term refers to the process of gradually increasing the automaticity of practiced strategies, which facilitates independence through the use of compensatory strategies and tools. As individuals learn to perform a task or skill, repetitive practice allows them to become more effective at compensating for their cognitive deficits with less reliance on external assistance. For example, after weeks of external reminders to check the next day's schedule before bed each night, this process becomes a part of an individual's nightly routine such that checking the schedule is initiated '"automatically" without external cueing.

Generalization: The process by which a patient learns to apply skills learned with one task or in one setting to a variety of other similar tasks or settings. The goal is to enable the patient to apply appropriate strategies for managing deficits in personally relevant areas of everyday functioning. For example, once the memory book is mastered for use with tracking appointments, usage can be transferred to another functional area such as tracking household chores.

1.5 Process and Flow of Therapy

1.5.a Overall Stages of Treatment

Treatment takes place in two phases. The first phase includes comprehensive assessment and rehabilitation planning. The second phase involves implementing the treatment plan.

A comprehensive neuropsychological assessment should in most cases be completed to identify the underlying cognitive and/or neurobehavioral impairments that interfere with effective daily functioning, as well as those relative strengths that support functioning and can be engaged to assist necessary use of compensatory strategies.

The neuropsychological assessment can provide an invaluable guide to treatment, not only by identifying areas of deficit, but by showing how deficits in one area will impact treatment in another. For example, training in the use of a Memory Notebook may be compromised by other deficits in executive functioning, which impede planning and organizing information. By the same token, training in executive functions may be affected by underlying deficits in attention and concentration. For this reason, it will be important to identify all areas of cognitive impairment and to develop a coordinated plan to address each one. The neuropsychological examination will also help the rehabilitation team identify the emotional and psychological struggles the patient may be experiencing, and help guide the cognitive rehabilitation process.

Once problems and priorities are identified, the therapist determines the tasks or environments in which the impairment interferes with functioning (e.g., vocational tasks, home management). Then, strategies are chosen to address the issue, and activities are selected that will improve the patient's daily functioning within that domain. Chosen tasks should be both relevant to the patient's life and reflect the underlying cognitive deficit, even if the goal is to improve performance on a specific task without the expectation that the skills learned will generalize to other tasks or settings. For example, a patient with memory impairment might employ strategies to navigate to the local community center for daily activities, and this strategy may or may not generalize to other destinations in which navigational or memory impairment may be a challenge. Finally, this phase requires deciding where treatment will be carried out, whether the focus will be limited to a specific task or environment, or if the goal is to address behavior across a variety of settings. The information gathered during this phase is then used to develop an individualized treatment plan.

In the second phase of treatment, the treatment plan is carried out as the patient learns the treatment strategies and begins to apply them. This takes place in three hierarchical stages (See Table 1-1): Acquisition, Application and Adaptation (Sohlberg & Mateer, 2001).

Table 1-1   Treatment Goals and Strategies Associated with Each Stage of Cognitive Rehabilitation

STAGE OF TREATMENT	GOALS	TYPE OF STRATEGIES USED
Acquisition	1) Teach purpose and procedures of treatment model. 2) Help patient recognize and accept deficits and benefits of treatment.	External
Application	1) Improve effectiveness and independence in compensating for deficits. 2) Promote internalization of strategies.	1) External 2) Internal
Adaptation	1) Promote transfer of training to tasks including those that are less structured, more novel, complex, and/or distracting. 2) Promote generalization of skills from the structured therapy setting to less structured environments such as home, community, and work.	1) External and Internal 2) External and Internal

Acquisition Stage

In the acquisition stage, patients are taught the various features of the chosen treatment strategy. They learn the purpose and procedures of the particular model to be used in treatment, and become familiar with any relevant supporting materials such as a notebook, worksheets, or other tools. Problem orientation and awareness is also addressed at this stage to help patients learn to recognize the nature of the behavioral or cognitive problems they are having, and to understand the rationale and benefits of receiving treatment. Something as simple as recording performance in a particular task with and without strategy use can facilitate awareness of the need for compensations.

In many cases, upon completion of this phase, the patient will be able to recall explicitly the steps involved in the procedure and explain the reason why each is important. In other cases, individuals may rely on procedural learning (e.g., use an external cue as a trigger for initiating an appropriate response), even if they cannot describe what they are doing.

Application Stage

Patients begin to apply the strategy to simple tasks, often in the context of their therapy sessions or in-clinic activities in the application stage. Usually this process begins with a high level of external support and supervision (e.g., therapist demonstration, verbal instruction, modeling, coaching, overt guidance). The therapist's role is to provide cues and assistance to help facilitate the patient's performance, review the patient's work, and provide constructive feedback to help the patient master the use of the strategy. The focus of rehabilitation may evolve to promote internalization and reduced reliance on external cues if the patient becomes able to use the strategy independently using external cues (e.g., following instruction sheets, using cue cards). This transition is begun by providing ample practice and gradual removal of external cues to help the patient learn to apply the strategy using self-generated, internal cues. For those unable to use a strategy independently, the goal of therapy is to promote procedural learning. Here, the therapist provides ample structure, practice, and repetition to help maximize the patient's ability to use external aids effectively to perform simple, rote functional tasks.

Adaptation Stage

The patient begins to apply the strategy to more functional and everyday tasks outside the clinic or structured treatment environment in the adaptation stage. Target tasks can include any of the basic or more complex activities of daily living, such as medication management, money management, and cooking. The emphasis at this stage is on promoting generalization by teaching patients how to apply successfully the skills they have learned to a broader range of tasks and environments, including those that are more unstructured, novel, complex, and/or distracting. In general, any task that was previously performed in the structured therapy environment is now attempted outside the therapy environment or in the community. Structured homework assignments in which a patient records their activity to allow in-session feedback provides an excellent means of facilitating adaptation of strategies as well as promoting active patient participation in the therapy process.

Although treatment should focus on promoting generalization whenever possible, some patients will not be able to apply learned strategies or procedures independently in other settings (generalization) or on other similar tasks (transfer of training). Generalization requires that the patient has the ability to recognize similarities between the situation in which the skill was learned and situations that they encounter later on. For many patients, particularly those with significant deficits in executive functions such as concept formation, cognitive flexibility, abstract reasoning, and self-monitoring, the ability to generalize can be limited. For those patients who are unable to generalize learned strategies to novel contexts, external cueing will be necessary for optimal functioning.

Cognitive rehabilitation requires systematic and ongoing data collection on the patient's performance. Appendix B provides forms that can be utilized for this purpose. Systematic data collection provides for a consistent measurement of progress which patients often find meaningful. Consistent feedback regarding their progress sustains their engagement in therapy and provides objective data that they are reaching rehabilitation goals. Graphs derived from the data collected from the forms in Appendix B are particularly useful not only for the patient, but for families and reimbursement sources as well.

1.6   External Versus Internal Strategies

The BI-ISIG recommendations reflect treatment strategies that refer to the global plan and method chosen to address a particular problem. These strategies can be external or internal. *External* strategies are those that are external to the patient, including the use of notebooks and other written planning systems, electronic devices, computerized systems, auditory or visual cueing systems, and task-specific aids (such as Post-it® notes, cue cards, pocket notebooks, home calendars, etc.). The long-term goal of these procedures is to enable patients to compensate for their impairments independently by using aids to assist them in performing daily functional, household, vocational, or work-related tasks (Sohlberg & Mateer, 2001). *Internal* strategies, on the other hand, include any self-generated procedure whose purpose is to enhance conscious control over one's thoughts, behaviors, or emotions. This is achieved by teaching patients to cue themselves to use an image, word, or action sequence as a trigger to take the appropriate steps to address a task or problem at hand. The long-term goal of these strategies is to enable patients to become so familiar with the process and adept at using it, that they can use it in any situation, even without external assistance.

In the early stages of treatment, strategies are typically not self-generated and the therapist provides the patient with instructions and guidelines which are, by definition, external. The patient's task is simply to follow the directions and use the strategy to complete the particular task. As rehabilitation progresses, the therapist can incorporate the use of both external and internal strategies.

While specific treatment strategies and procedures will vary depending on both the patient's abilities and the domain being addressed, the treatment process typically starts by providing a high level of external structure, guidance, and support to assist the patient. The patient's ability to use external strategies independently under highly structured and supervised circumstances will determine whether a shift in treatment is appropriate. As the patient becomes more effective at implementing external strategies without external supervision and assistance, treatment begins to incorporate the use of internal strategies as well. In this case, the amount of structure is gradually withdrawn until the patient can independently remember and use the internal strategy when necessary through self-cuing.

An example of shifting from external to internal strategy use might include teaching the patient how to use self-talk by whispering to oneself the steps of a procedure that were previously provided in writing or with verbal prompts (Miechenbaum & Goodman, 1971). Thus, what started out external eventually becomes internal (Cicerone & Wood, 1987). Even for those patients with milder problems, this process of internalization requires a great deal of practice. Over time, strategy use may become automatic, but even if this occurs, ideally the patient remains capable of controlling its use.

Four levels of outcome are possible, depending on the patient's progress:

1) The patient never develops the necessary awareness or motivation to become independent in compensating for his/her deficits. Therefore, the patient only learns to perform simple routines and action sequences procedurally.

2) The patient learns independent use of external aids to compensate; he/she can perform some things internally, but still needs some external guidance.

3) The patient is able to internalize fully-learned strategies and can independently self-generate and apply these strategies without external assistance or aids in specific situations and/or tasks.

4) The patient is able to generalize learned skills to a range of situations and/or tasks.

1.7   A Guide to Treatment Planning and (Tactical) Goal Writing

Ideally, treatment planning and goal setting is a collaborative process with the patient and/or their family playing an integral role in helping develop appropriate and personally relevant goals. Often patients want to know when they can resume previous life roles, responsibilities, and activities such as returning to school, work, and driving. However, especially early on in treatment, it is not always possible to answer these questions. Because of the difficulties in reliably predicting recovery, it is important for the therapist to try to strike a balance between fostering hopefulness while also helping patients evaluate their progress on rehabilitation goals to determine if their long-term outcome goals can be achieved. Objective measurement of progress on short-term tactical goals, collaborative appraisal of progress, and constructive counseling are very important to assist the patient in modifying goals as necessary, as well as to sustain motivation and engagement in the therapeutic process. Once long-term goals are identified (e.g., going back to school), the therapist helps break them down into a series of shorter-term goals that are measurable.

It is essential that the patient understand the connection or relevance of therapeutic tasks to their long-term goals; no one is motivated to engage in behavior they find irrelevant. Big goals (e.g., going back to driving) are best addressed as a series of gradual steps, with each step regarded as an experiment that might fail. As a general rule, when a patient is making good progress, it is reasonable to expect more progress. Alternatively, when a patient no longer is making progress, it is very important to consider consultation from other rehabilitation professionals, and consider alternative treatment strategies. Some therapists, particularly novice or beginner therapists, may perceive a lack of progress as threatening to their own self-esteem. In some cases, this can cause a therapist to either withdraw emotionally from the patient or project blame on the patient for not making progress. It can be difficult to remain patient and engaged, as cognitive rehabilitation can be a slow process. Potential reasons for a lack of progress are many, but often include the patient's understanding of the relationship between short-term therapeutic goals and their long-term outcome goals (e.g., returning to work), how progress is measured, the selection of therapeutic tasks, or the patient's psychological status.

1.7.a   Moving from Strategies to Tactics

A good treatment plan begins by first determining the best strategy for addressing the problem. In this manual, the term *strategies* refers to the broad, general therapeutic approach taken to address a cognitive impairment or functional limitation. Some strategies have been noted in the BI-ISIG recommendations. Thus, someone with a severe memory problem may be treated with the overall *strategy* of using a Memory Notebook system to record and retain information.

However, once a strategy is selected, the therapist must decide on how to implement it. Strategy implementation is achieved through a series of tactics designed to help the patient achieve the desired outcome. This implementation is the tactical dimension. *Tactics*, in this case, involve the specific tasks the patient is asked to perform (e.g., using a notebook to schedule simple household tasks), as well as the measures used to evaluate success (e.g., the amount of external assistance required for the patient to use the notebook strategy effectively).

In this manual, we provide a model for treatment planning and goal setting that captures as complete a picture as possible of a patient's deficits, and the strategies and tactics used to address them. The specific BI-ISIG recommendations for each of the deficit areas, along with an accompanying list of associated treatment strategies, tactics, and sample goals can be found in Appendix A. It is our hope that the practice of writing goals in as detailed a manner as possible will provide a clear framework to guide the course of rehabilitation and facilitate the measurement of progress using the templates found in Appendix B.

1.7.b   Long-Term (strategic) and Short-Term (tactical) Goals

In global terms, rehabilitation goals tend to be either *long-term* or *short-term*. By their nature, treatment strategies reflect a broader, long-term treatment effort, while it is expected that implementing and evaluating the success of particular treatment tactics will be accomplished over a much shorter period of time. Accordingly, when writing goals in rehabilitation settings, it is important to take into consideration the length of time it will take a patient to achieve them. In addition, because of the shorter time frame allotted for each, short-term (tactical) goals are typically more specific than long-term (strategic) goals. For example, a patient with memory problems might have a strategic long-term goal to "improve ability to independently compensate for memory deficits using external aids," whereas the corresponding short-term tactical goal might be "patient will initiate simple household tasks in a timely manner with minimal assistance using a Memory Notebook strategy."

1.7.c   Anatomy of a Short-Term Goal

In rehabilitation settings, patients' progress, usually measured at the tactical level, is evaluated on a regular (i.e., daily, weekly or biweekly) basis. This provides an effective and quantifiable means of monitoring the patient's progress, and facilitates determination of whether the chosen tactics are effective. This process also encourages ongoing assessment of whether current goals are appropriate, or if they need to be modified to better reflect tangible progress and maintain patient motivation for treatment. Several factors are involved in writing short-term (i.e., tactical) goals for cognitive rehabilitation, including task variables (type of task, complexity of task), measures of success (percentage of accurate responses, speed to completion, level of assistance needed, and the various strategies that a given patient may be asked to use).

Accordingly, a comprehensive template for goal-writing might include the following five factors:

1) Type of task
2) Complexity of the task
3) Level of cueing or assistance needed
4) Type of strategy employed
5) Measure of success (e.g., speed, accuracy)

So, using our earlier example of memory book training: Patient will perform *simple* **(2)**; *household tasks that require scheduling* **(1)**; *with minimal assistance* **(3)**; to use a *memory notebook strategy* **(4)**; and at *100% accuracy* **(5)**.

There are, of course, a number of ways in which a comprehensive tactical goal might be written, both in terms of style and content, and not every goal will need to reflect each of the five factors.

Table 1-2 provides an outline of the five factors that comprise a comprehensive tactical goal, along with examples of each.

Table 1-2   Factors that Comprise a Comprehensive Short-Term Goal

STAGE OF TREATMENT	GOALS
1) Type of task	Impairment level tasks: » Divided attention tasks » Problem-solving/reasoning tasks » Sequencing tasks » Memory tasks » Organization tasks » Planning tasks » Flexibility tasks Functional tasks: » Clinic tasks (e.g., carrying out daily treatment schedule) » Self care or instrumental activities of daily living (ADL) tasks (e.g., dressing, money management, medication management) » Household tasks (e.g., cooking, laundry, cleaning) » Community tasks (e.g., shopping, community travel) » Work-related tasks (e.g., filing, computer data entry)
2) Complexity of the task	» Simple » Moderate » Complex
3) Level of cueing or assistance needed	» None » Mild » Moderate » Maximum
4) Type of strategy employed	Examples of external strategies include: » Memory notebook » Electronic memory device (e.g., pager, Cadex watch, digital timer, smart/cell phones) » Task-specific aids (e.g., Post-it® notes, cue cards, pocket notebooks, home calendars) Examples of internal strategies include: » Problem-solving procedures (e.g., Goal Management Training) » Neglect protocols (e.g., The Lighthouse Strategy) » Time Pressure Management Training » Self instructional strategies (e.g., Self Monitoring Training, Cognitive Behavioral and other self-talk strategies) » Internal memory strategies (e.g., mnemonics, visual imagery)
5) Measure of success (e.g., speed, accuracy)	» Percentage of accurate responses » Speed to complete task » Level of cuing or assistance needed; this can range from maximal assistance to none

1.7.d Sample Template for Goal Setting

In Appendix A, a comprehensive list of long-term (strategic) goals and the accompanying short-term (tactical) goals is provided. Sample treatment plan templates are also included to facilitate the writing of both strategic and tactical goals. Because each person with a brain injury is unique in his or her presentation, goals, and needs, the treatment planning process is highly individualized. To determine the starting point for goal setting with a particular patient, baseline measures should be obtained, such as task speed/accuracy, patient awareness, and level of cueing or assistance required for the patient to perform the desired task and/or compensate for the target impairment. Careful observation of the patient's emotional reaction to the task is very important as well. These reactions can often guide the observant therapist's presentation of tasks as well as the interpersonal context in which they occur.

Below is a completed sample treatment plan that outlines a treatment for memory impairments with notebook training. It is based on the following BI-ISIG recommendations:

BI-ISIG Committee Recommendations

Practice Standard: For individuals with mild impairment, the committee recommends the use of internalized strategies (e.g., mnemonics, visual imagery) and external memory compensations (e.g., notebooks, electronic devices).

Practice Guideline: For individuals with moderate to severe impairment, the committee recommends only the use of external compensations (including notebooks, electronic devices, etc.) with direct application to functional activities.

Long-Term (strategic) Goal – Effectively use external aids to compensate for memory deficits during daily activities. Anticipated time frame – 3 months.

Month 1: **Strategic Monthly Goal**

1) Implement Acquisition stage of Memory Notebook training.

Short-term (tactical) Goals

1) Patient will recall simple autobiographical information with maximum cues to use Memory Notebook with 75% accuracy.

2) Patient will perform simple household tasks that require scheduling with maximal cues to initiate use of Memory Notebook strategy with 75% accuracy.

Month 2: **Strategic Monthly Goal**

1) Initiate Application stage of memory notebook training.

Short-term (tactical) Goals

1) Patient will answer questions re: personal history with minimal cues using a memory book strategy with 100% accuracy.

2) Patient will perform simple household tasks requiring scheduling with minimal cues using a Memory Notebook strategy with 100% accuracy.

Month 3: **Strategic Monthly Goal**

1) Complete Application stage of memory book training.

Short-term (tactical) Goals

1) Patient will carry out daily treatment schedule with independent use of memory book at 100% accuracy.

2) Patient will perform semi-complex household tasks requiring scheduling with independent use of Memory Notebook and 75% accuracy.

1.8 Treatment Considerations When Designing Training Procedures

1.8.a Task-Specific versus Strategic Approaches to Treatment

Depending on their purpose, protocols can be designed to improve performance on a specific task (e.g., self-administering medications), or they can be broad and aimed at improving performance or compensating for an overall domain of impairment (e.g., memory). In contrast with task-specific approaches, which are aimed at the functional level, strategies emphasize the utilization of cognitive process or system (strategy), in context of performing functional tasks, through which the patient can overcome the effects of an impairment of cognitive functioning.

Research seems to support a strategic approach to treatment because, by offering a means to compensate for existing cognitive deficits, there is a better likelihood of generalization outside the treatment setting. A task-specific approach may result in the acquisition of skills necessary to perform a particular task or routine. However, for an intervention to be effective in the long-term, patients need to be able to transfer learned skills to a range of daily tasks and situations (Ownsworth & McFarland, 1999). As will be discussed in the following sections, there are times when a strategic approach may not be appropriate. In these cases, where the emphasis is on maximizing procedural learning, a task-specific approach may be more appropriate.

1.8.b External versus Internal Strategies

To use a strategy independently, one needs to have some capacity to internalize it, i.e., to develop some conscious control over its use. However, not all patients are capable of internalization, in which case a more external strategy may be the only option.

As a general guideline, those patients with mild impairment can benefit from both external and internal approaches and strategies. However, while the use of internal strategies (e.g., memory mnemonics) may be appropriate for those with mild to moderate impairment, patients with more severe impairments in memory, self-awareness, or overall cognitive functioning tend to do best with external (i.e., procedural) strategies. The essential goal is to provide enough practice to eventuate performance to a level of automaticity. In that case, it will be unconscious, controlled by habit, and not deliberately directed. The patient will learn to produce the desired response, but without the benefit of insight or self-management. This approach is best suited for treatments aimed at improving performance on specific tasks or routines.

The decision regarding which external device to use in any given situation involves a number of factors, including: (1) the particular task that the patient wishes to perform; (2) the patient's goals, abilities, disabilities and preferences; (3) the access to and availability of technology; and (4) the environment in which technology is going to be used (Sohlberg & Mateer, 2001). Figure 1-1 provides a decision tree outlining the general options in treatment planning for cognitive rehabilitation.

Figure 1-1: Decision Tree for Treatment Planning

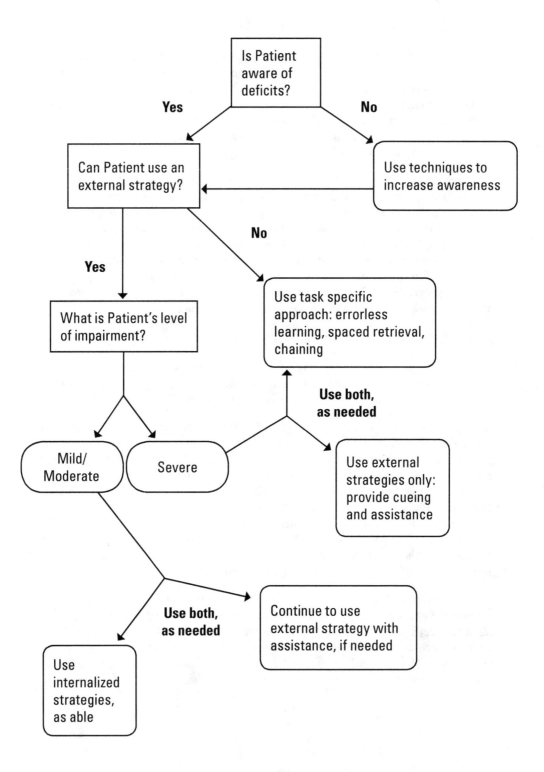

1.9 Neurobehavioral and Psychosocial Factors that Influence Treatment Process and Outcome

1.9.a Patient Variables

A variety of injury-specific factors affect the priorities and process of cognitive rehabilitation. Perhaps even more important, however, is the human, individual context in which the impairment occurs. The values and priorities of patients, their history in dealing with stressful circumstances, and their sense of self-worth and self-efficacy can all have a significant effect on their reaction to efforts to rehabilitate impairments of cognitve functioning. The patient's emotional reaction not only to their impairments, but also to the frequent daily confrontations with the effects of their impairments, need to be incorporated into the execution of each therapeutic encounter.

Impairments of Awareness

There is a broad consensus that unawareness of one's impairments has a significant impact on treatment outcomes. Those with less insight or awareness will have less motivation to engage fully in treatment and, as a result, will require more structure and assistance to learn strategies and apply them to their day-to-day functioning. The treatment of unawareness is addressed in Section 2.7 Metacognitive Strategy Training for Behavioral and Emotional Dysregulation.

Typically, treatment begins with an assessment of the presence and nature of impairments of awareness. The assessment of awareness is important because there are different causes for impairments of awareness, and these differences have a significant impact on how the impairment of awareness is managed. There are three major causes of awareness deficits: (1) neurocognitive factors; (2) psychological factors; and (3) social/environmental factors (Fleming & Ownsworth, 2006).

Neurocognitive unawareness, or "anosognosia," is common in those patients with moderate to severe brain damage. There are two variants or subtypes within the category of neurocognitive unawareness: global and specific. Globally impaired patients are those whose brain damage is frontal and/or diffuse. They typically show unawareness that derives from underlying difficulties with reasoning and abstract thought. In this case, unawareness reflects an underlying inability to generalize, i.e., to draw general conclusions from specific items of information.

Accordingly, patients must be able to look at their own responses and recognize that they are incorrect. In effect, they must use reasoning to infer that they have made mistakes. In addition, they must use reasoning to infer that the mistakes they make indicate the presence of an underlying cognitive impairment. Finally, they must use reasoning to infer that their cognitive impairment strongly suggests a problem with functional, everyday tasks. In effect, they proceed from, for example, "I make mistakes on many visuospatial tasks," to "Therefore, I must have a visuospatial impairment," to "Therefore, I may have trouble driving a car." All three areas of inference require the ability to reason and generalize from specific facts to general conclusions.

Another type of neurocognitive unawareness is domain-specific according to the location of injury. Patients with injury to the parietal lesions are particularly likely to be unaware of the associated cognitive impairments, such as aphasia for patients with left parietal damage and those with hemispatial neglect associated with right parietal damage. Although often capable of formal reasoning, the nature of their injuries makes it difficult for them to perceive and recognize their specific impairments.

Psychological denial can easily produce behaviors which appear to represent neuro-cognitive unawareness. Psychological denial is motivated by the need to ignore very emotionally painful thoughts that accompany the conscious recognition of a cognitive impairment. Premorbid personality traits (e.g., the use of denial and repression as defense mechanisms) can contribute to psychological unawareness, though varying levels of denial can also be seen in individuals who have yet to complete the normal process of grief, acceptance, and adjustment. It is emotionally difficult for people to accept a loss fully, and fostering a realistic sense of hope for continued recovery can facilitate adjustment.

Individual and/or family-based psychotherapy can help individuals work through issues of psychological unawareness and adjustment to disability. As is the case in most forms of therapy, a strong therapeutic alliance can serve as a foundation from which to work collaboratively on self-image, coping strategies, and acceptance of disability. Family therapy can be useful in helping a patient and his/her support network to adjust to new roles, discuss expectations, and establish cues and external supports to maximize generalization of learned strategies to the "real-world" environment.

The third type of unawareness stems from a general lack of information about brain injury and functional impairments. Some patients simply have not been told about their impairments, or have not engaged in the kind of tasks that would demonstrate the existence of these impairments. For example, if caretakers focus primarily on a patient's physical injuries during acute rehabilitation, cognitive changes might have been overlooked or minimized. Similarly, cognitive impairments may have been 'masked' during the early stages of recovery, and impairments may not be recognized until the patient attempts to return to work and realizes he or she is no longer capable of many required tasks. In other cases, patients may have been inadvertently encouraged or reinforced by well-intentioned family members to deny the existence of problems.

For patients with unawareness stemming from lack of information, individual and family education is the starting point to address the problem. Psychoeducation about brain injury and rehabilitation is often sufficient to raise awareness, and it can also serve to clarify misinformation, misunderstandings, and questions held by both patients and family members. Psychoeducation and feedback help to validate a patient's experiences by explaining that many of their symptoms are quite common after brain injury, and can also help family members to understand the reasons for some of the unusual behaviors that they have observed in their loved one. However, education is not always sufficient, particularly if a patient's behavior is disruptive or the family is defensive. In these cases, individual and/or family therapy may be indicated.

It is also important to note that some therapeutic interventions need to be avoided when working with certain types of unawareness. The therapist may need to avoid direct confrontation or attempts to educate the patient about their impairments when unawareness is psychologically motivated. Group therapy can be especially threatening for the patient with psychological denial unless they have a great deal of trust of other members and also experience a great deal of support and acceptance in the group. Many patients experience feelings of intense vulnerability when awareness of impairment begins to emerge, and even very subtle feedback or comments can easily be perceived by the patient to be confrontational and insensitive. In these cases, a series of private meetings with the patient, conducted in a collaborative manner, may be more helpful (Giacino & Cicerone, 1998).

Severity and Range of Impairment

Patients with severe deficits in attention, memory, or executive functioning may be unable to learn, remember, and use internal strategies, or to generalize the skills they have learned. As a general rule, if a patient demonstrates the capacity to learn, remember and exert conscious behavioral control, treatment should incorporate both a general approach and the use of internalized strategies whenever possible. Therefore, knowing the scope and severity of different domains of cognitive impairment can provide invaluable information to help guide treatment planning. As with any therapy, the severity of impairment will have a major impact on the level of structured cueing and assistance that the patient will need. It should also be noted that the severity of the injury itself (i.e., duration of loss of consciousness or post-traumatic amnesia.) is sometimes, but not always, predictive of the severity of longstanding functional impairment a patient might experience. Some individuals who have sustained severe injuries can experience remarkable recovery and have only mild residual impairments, while some individuals who have sustained relatively minor injuries can experience disabling impairment.

Emotional Reactions and Premorbid Psychiatric Issues

Alterations in mood, emotional regulation, and behavioral control are common consequences of brain injury. These issues may be the direct result of the neuropathological changes following brain injury, secondary to adjustment difficulties, related to preexisting psychological factors, or not uncommonly, related to an interaction of all three.

It makes intuitive sense that one's emotional state could affect both treatment participation and outcomes. Research supports the notion that patients who are depressed are less motivated for therapy (Robinson & Jorge, 1994). Likewise, poor coping skills or difficulties with anger management may intensify adjustment difficulties, while feelings of anxiety may limit one's willingness to attempt new and/or challenging tasks. Finally, those with premorbid psychiatric disorders may experience an exacerbation of symptoms such as behavioral withdrawal, depression, agitation, or paranoia. Thus, it is important to obtain a thorough history in addition to obtaining information about a patient's current level of emotional functioning. In cases where mood or emotional issues are prominent, it may be necessary to involve the support of a psychologist for therapy and/or a physician for psychopharmacologic intervention.

1.9.b   Family Factors

Although outside the scope of this manual, there are a few essential points worth mentioning with respect to the influence of family on the recovery process. It is important to recognize that brain injuries are events that profoundly impact the entire family, not just the survivor of the brain injury. The homeostasis within the family system is significantly disrupted by the trauma, often resulting in role changes, strained relationships, increased familial stress, as well as increased financial burden. All of these factors can impair family cohesiveness and drain coping skills. Throughout the rehabilitation and recovery process, the family will struggle to reorganize itself to adjust to changes in role identity and demands (Kay & Cavallo, 1994).

As a result of the significant impact these changes can have on the rehabilitation process, it is generally agreed that family collaboration can facilitate both recovery and treatment outcomes (Kay & Cavallo, 1994). Research suggests that integrating the family into treatment can enhance functional outcomes and, in fact, it can be pivotal to successful generalization outside of structured treatment settings to the home environment (Sohlberg & Mateer, 2001). At the very least, family members should be educated regarding the nature of patients' impairments, and how these impairments may impact on the family system. Prognosis and long-term care needs should also be discussed so caregivers can develop realistic expectations and plans with respect to their ability to manage the patient effectively in the community.

Although typically it is recommended and beneficial to integrate the family into treatment, there are times when a family member's contribution can disrupt the therapeutic process. Some examples include, but are not limited to, young children feeling uncomfortable seeing or interacting with the patient, family members inadvertently impeding progress by trying to do too much for the patient, or by not adhering to staff recommendations for maintaining safety precautions. These examples further underscore the benefit and importance of providing the family with psycho-education and psychotherapy to assist them in adapting to the ever-changing dynamic of recovery and the implications for their relationship and roles. Brain injury support groups, both in-person and through internet forums, can also provide important and invaluable resources to assist the family throughout the recovery process.

1.10   Monitoring Progress in Cognitive Rehabilitation

Keeping records of a patient's progress is strongly recommended to keep both the patient and the therapist focused on goals of treatment. Specific techniques and data forms will vary considerably across approaches to treatment, but two general rules of thumb should be adhered to when implementing cognitive rehabilitation after acquired brain injury.

The first is to create a detailed record of task performance during sessions to monitor a patient's successes and failures on specific tasks. An example of clinically useful data recording forms can be found in Appendix B. This data-driven approach serves the purpose of creating an objective record of performance, which can help a patient and therapist to identify factors that enhance or reduce successful outcomes. For example, during attention training, a therapist might record the number of errors made on each attention task, as recommended by Sohlberg and Mateer (1987b). A therapist should also make note of what strategies a patient was using during each task, or what internal or external distractions arose during the task. Data on errors is not particularly useful in the absence of data that can help to explain variations in performance. When objective data demonstrates that using a particular strategy enhances performance, motivation to use this strategy may be increased. Similarly, when performance declines in the presence of external distractions (e.g., noise in the hallway), environmental compensations can be implemented to maximize performance (e.g., turning off the television when making a phone call). Detailed records of in-session task performance can also help to raise a patient's awareness of how factors such as fatigue can influence their cognitive abilities. If performance declines after several trials, this may indicate that fatigue is impacting performance and a break is needed. A patient can use this data to help develop an in-the-moment awareness of how and when fatigue begins to impact performance so that a break can be initiated. Finally, detailed session records can help the therapist to plan the next session, tailor or tweak strategy training, and modify treatment goals.

The second general rule of thumb is to keep track of "big picture" progress. Cognitive rehabilitation can be a very long and challenging process, and many patients have a hard time recognizing the progress they have made. Helping a patient to identify and record personally relevant milestones, a log or journal can facilitate motivation and instill hope. These records can be reviewed periodically throughout treatment in order to recognize and celebrate changes that may otherwise be overlooked. Many patients will at times feel overwhelmed by their deficits, and it can be encouraging to look at data that shows progress. It can be stressful for patients to think about the things they can't do, and patients should be encouraged to give themselves credit for the progress they've made. (e.g., "When we first started working together your mother brought you to the clinic because you couldn't travel alone. Now you take the train here independently.") It may sometimes be necessary for therapists and/or family members to keep track of a patient's functional gains, particularly when a patient does not have sufficient awareness or insight to recognize improvements.

2. Rehabilitation For Impairments of Executive Functions

2.1 Introduction

The term "executive functioning" refers to integrative cognitive processes that determine goal-directed and purposeful behavior. Executive functions are superordinate to more basic cognitive processes such as memory and attention. By supervising and coordinating underlying cognitive, behavioral, and emotional processes, executive functions allow for the orderly execution of daily life functions. These integrative functions include the ability to formulate goals, solve problems, anticipate the consequences of actions, plan and organize behavior, initiate relevant behaviors, and monitor and adapt behavior to fit a particular task or context. Disturbances of executive functions are also related to impaired emotional and behavioral self-regulation, and metacognitive processes (e.g., self-monitoring, error awareness and correction, and capacity for insight) (Cicerone et al., 2000).

A disturbance of executive functioning is most likely to be evident in novel or unfamiliar situations (Godefroy & Rousseaux, 1997). Executive functions are necessary to adapt to deviations from an established routine, react to unexpected events, or correct mistakes. Remedial interventions for acquired cognitive impairments often emphasize the acquisition of specific compensations in controlled situations. Rehabilitation of executive functions is necessary to teach metacognitive skills that can be applied across diverse situations.

Responsibility for the selection and application of compensatory strategies may initially rely on the therapist, with the hope that the patient will eventually be capable of implementing these compensations independently with adequate practice. Disturbances of executive functioning may limit the extent to which a patient is able to participate actively in the selection and application of compensatory strategies, at least initially. Choosing and applying the appropriate compensations requires some degree of intact awareness—both self-awareness and situational awareness—which may be compromised after TBI.

2.2 Impairments of Executive Functions and Brain Dysfunction

Brain injury often results in deficits in executive functions. These can manifest as problems with self-directed cognitive functioning or they can manifest as problems with self-directed behavioral and emotional self-control, as described below.

Cognitively, individuals with executive dysfunction may find it difficult to think abstractly. These individuals usually have problems with awareness, anticipating problems, analyzing situations, planning solutions and executing those solutions, maintaining a flexible or pragmatic approach to tasks, and monitoring themselves (i.e., identifying and correcting errors, incorporating feedback from others).

In the emotional realm, executive dysfunction can result from damage to those areas of the brain that are responsible for inhibiting the limbic system and the direct expression of emotions. This can result in a loss or decrease in the ability to regulate and control one's emotions, which can cause a person to feel more extreme or quickly changing emotional highs or lows (emotional lability), or to become overwhelmed when experiencing emotions. These deficits stem from underlying brain dysfunction, which distinguishes them from those reactions that reflect a purely emotional reaction to perceived impairment, i.e., reactions that could be expected in many people even without brain dysfunction such as grief, sadness, anxiety, or frustration. Moreover, the nature of the underlying brain dysfunction distinguishes these emotional reactions from those seen secondary to mental illness and psychiatric disorders.

In the behavioral realm, patients with brain injury and executive dysfunction often fail to think before they act and show corresponding impulsivity, disinhibition, hyperverbosity, poor emotional control, and cognitive inflexibility. These "positive symptoms" are indications of behavior that is "stimulus-bound" or overly determined by the environment.

Although executive dysfunction commonly causes these "excessive" thoughts, emotions, and behaviors, executive dysfunction can also manifest as more "negative" symptoms that almost seem to be the opposite of those described above. These can include difficulty initiating tasks, low drive or motivation, apathy, impersistence, or aspontaneity. This constellation of symptoms is sometimes called adynamia.

It is important to note that both positive symptoms (disorders of excess) and negative symptoms (adynamia) can be present in the same individual and reflect a fundamental disturbance of self-regulation of thinking, feeling, and behavior (Cicerone and Giacino, 1992).

Medications, such as antidepressant or mood stabilizers, may reduce the intensity of neurobehavioral problems. However, in the context of brain injury rehabilitation, these problems can also be approached behaviorally by means of either external or internal strategies. Among the external strategies are behavioral modification and reinforcement, token economy, and environmental constraints. All of these require others to structure interventions with the patient. Internal strategies, in contrast, are those that are employed and managed by the patients themselves.

2.3 BI-ISIG Recommendations for Impairments of Executive Functions

The BI-ISIG Cognitive Rehabilitation Task Force of ACRM (Cicerone, et al. 2011) recommends, as a Practice Standard, metacognitive strategy training (self-monitoring and self-regulation) for deficits in executive functioning after TBI, including impairments of emotional self-regulation, and as a component of interventions for deficits in attention, neglect and memory.

The BI-ISIG also recommends, as a Practice Guideline, training in formal problem-solving strategies and their application to everyday situations and functional activities during post-acute rehabilitation after TBI. Problem-solving strategies are used to teach patients to approach situations in a rational and systematic fashion, analyze problems, consider alternate solutions, prioritize and execute a solution, and review the outcome.

The BI-ISIG also notes, as a Practice Option, that group-based interventions may be considered for remediation of executive and problem-solving deficits after TBI (Cicerone et al., 2011).

2.4 A General Framework for Rehabilitation of Impairments of Executive Functions

The various interventions that have been developed for executive dysfunction attempt to reinforce the use of conscious and deliberate strategies to re-establish external structure and/or improve a patient's ability to exercise control over his/her behavior. Most interventions in this area follow a common approach, which parallels the structure of executive functioning: the creation of a structured plan that leads to a desired outcome; execution of a response or sequence of responses; and the use of feedback to compare the structured plan with the achieved outcome, and modification of one's plan accordingly (Miller, Galanter & Pribram, 1960; Teuber, 1964).

Prior to initiating a given task, the patient is instructed to identify the demands associated with the task, and to plan the appropriate sequence of responses. In some cases, patients may be asked to predict explicitly the expected outcome of their behavior. This allows for comparison of expected and observed outcomes, an activity that can facilitate awareness and improve self-monitoring.

Next, the person implements his/her plan to perform the task, actively self-monitors performance and use of strategies throughout. The therapist should determine the amount of structure and cueing provided at this level of intervention to facilitate on-line monitoring (e.g. awareness and correction of errors) and strategy application.

Finally the person compares the effectiveness of their actions with the predicted effects and consequences, and evaluates their performance (typically while incorporating feedback from the therapist and/or others). While the specific language and aspects of interventions represented in this section will vary, this structure and process is common to most metacognitive and problem-solving interventions for impairments of executive functioning and can serve as framework for understanding and implementing these various interventions (see Tables 2-1 and 2-2, below).

This sequence provides a general algorithm for rehabilitation of executive dysfunction involving (1) anticipation and planning of potential responses to novel tasks or problem-solving situations; (2) implementation and self-monitoring of selected responses; and (3) evaluation of the outcome of the response, comparing the outcome with the desired or anticipated outcome, and changing the approach to the task, if necessary, which then "resets" the sequence of operations. The application of this algorithm to a number of specific metacognitive strategies is shown in Table 2-1 and the relationship of this algorithm to several problem-solving strategies is shown in Table 2-2.

In clinical practice, the sequence above is often preceded by attempts to assess and foster the patient's awareness of deficits, identifying the relevant strategies and setting goals. Crosson et al. (1989) have described a useful framework for understanding impaired self-awareness after TBI that aligns each level of awareness with appropriate treatment approaches. Intellectual awareness refers to the basic acknowledgement of deficits resulting from illness or injury. This level of awareness requires the person to implement compensations routinely in all situations. Emergent awareness refers to the recognition of deficits in the course of actual functioning, and enables the person to implement compensations once the potential impact of a deficit is recognized.

These two levels of awareness, intellectual and emergent, parallel the distinction between self-knowledge (i.e., general self-awareness and beliefs about one's abilities) and on-line awareness (i.e., task-specific awareness that is activated in specific situations or during performance of an activity) (Goverover et al., 2007; Toglia & Kirk, 2000). The third level of awareness, anticipatory awareness, refers to the person's ability to anticipate the potential impact of one's deficits or aspects of a situation on performance, and therefore anticipate the need for a compensatory strategy. Setting an appropriate goal and selection of relevant strategies may vary depending on the level of self-awareness.

The decision regarding which strategy to use with a given patient will, in large part, be determined by the severity of the patient's injuries and the degree of executive dysfunction associated with those injuries. As will be discussed below, recommended strategies for individuals with severe impairment will tend to differ considerably from those recommended for milder impairments. Figure 2-1 provides a decision tree for treatment planning for impairments of executive functions.

Figure 2-1 A Decision Tree for Treatment Planning for Executive Dysfunction

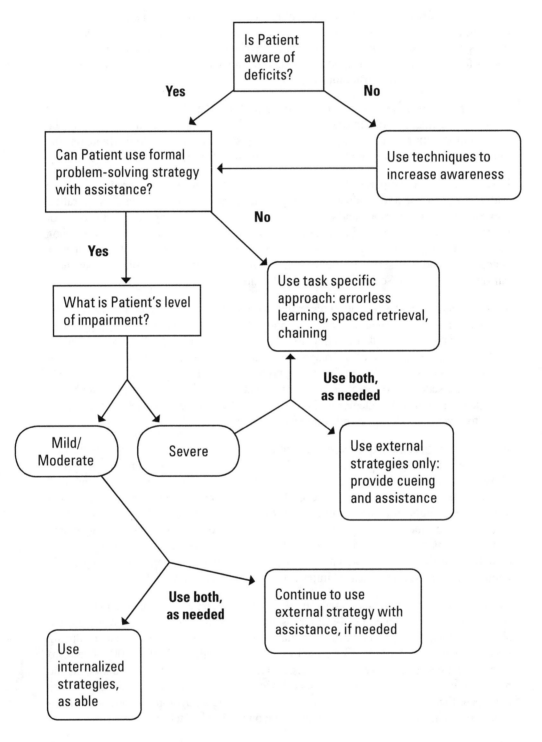

The protocols to be discussed in this section include: a protocol for formal problem-solving; a protocol for metacognitive techniques to address cognitive impairment; specific metacognitive techniques to address behavioral and emotional self-regulation; and finally, a list of complex programs to address executive function will be provided.

2.5 Metacognitive Strategy Training for Impairments of Executive Functions

Metacognition refers to "thinking about thinking" which includes both metacognitive knowledge and metacognitive control (Kennedy et al., 2008). Metacognitive knowledge represents both the person's moment-to-moment awareness of his or her thinking and more stable beliefs about one's cognitive abilities. Metacognitive control represents the person's self-monitoring of their thinking and the ability to adapt to changes in the environment or task-demands. Highly complex behaviors are products of self regulation or an executive function system that supports a set of skills that include (1) setting goals; (2) comparing performance with goals or outcomes; (3) making decisions to change one's behavior or select an alternative approach to a situation; and (4) executing the change in behavior. (Kennedy et al., 2008). These metacognitive processes are superordinate to, and influence, cognitive processes such as attention, comprehension, and memory.

Interventions directed at restoring these metacognitive processes are often refered to as "metacognitive strategy training." Although this is often discussed in relation to the treatment of executive dysfunction, these same strategies may be used to improve the persons's ability to pay attention, monitor their comprehension, improve their memory, or to improve other discrete skills.

Metacognitive strategy training is an umbrella term that applies to many top-down interventions. These should be distinguished from the more restorative/bottom-up interventions described in other sections.

Table 2-1 General Framework for Rehabilitation of Executive Deficits: Metacognitive Strategy Training

Intervention (Reference)	Awareness Intervention Protocol (Cheng & Man, 2006)	Self Awareness Training (Goverover et al., 2007)	Time Pressure Management (Winkens et al., 2009)

Awareness	Awareness of knowledge about deficits	General self-awareness of abilities
		
		On-line awareness
			Enhance the patient's awareness that mental slowness is a critical problem
			
			• Many activities affected by slowed speed
			   • Associated problems
			   • Fatigue
			   • Forgetfulness
			   • Emotional reactions

Anticipate / Plan	Predict performance on a functional task	Define task performance goals Predict task performance Anticipate and plan for errors or obstacles	Time Pressure Management Strategy ("Let me give myself enough time to do the Task") • Are there two or more things to be done at the same time? • Could I be overwhelmed or distracted? • Which things can be done before the actual task begins? Make a Plan • Do one thing at a time • Finish what I start
Execute / Self–Monitor	Perform task Monitor performance	Choose a strategy to circumvent difficulties Assess the assistance needed Perform IADL task	Monitor self while using TPM strategy. What to do in the case of unexpected time pressure? • Make an emergency plan • Plan and emergency plan ready? • Use Plan regularly
Self-Evaluate	Feedback given Self-evaluation Set short-term goals	Self-assess performance Therapist feedback Journal of experience	Generalization • Varied tasks • Varied level of difficulty • Varied level of distractions

In this section, we describe metacognitive strategies that are under the control and direction of self-generated cognitive processes, including the cueing, structure, and execution involved in the strategy. The goal of metacognitive strategy training and internalized strategies is to develop and enhance executive control over one's behaviors and the cognitive functions that support or inhibit them. Toward this end, the therapist attempts to remove obstacles that interfere with this self-control. These obstacles can be cognitive, emotional, or behavioral. Often they comprise all three.

The following is a review of the sub-processes involved in the treatment of cognitive and behavioral dysregulation, based on the problem-solving model described earlier. We will address the metacognitive treatment of problem-solving deficits first, followed by the metacognitive treatment of behavioral and emotional dysregulation.

2.5.a Metacognitive Strategy Training for Impairments in the Treatment of Executive Functioning Deficits

Although the primary goal of metacognitive training is to enhance a patient's ability to internalize awareness and control over his or her behavior, treatment typically begins with external cueing of a general rule or principle for solving problems. Accordingly, patients are taught the processes of self-monitoring and self-control by means of education, modeling, external directions, instructional handouts, and cueing. The specific procedure is of less importance than the fact that it contains all the elements that have been empirically validated.

Over time, through practice and implementation in a variety of settings, this external strategy can become internalized, under the self-generated direction of the patient. In essence, what begins as an external strategy becomes an internal strategy.

Metacognitive strategies may be relatively simple or complex. A simple strategy will be appropriate for those patients with moderate to severe impairment, e.g., training a patient in the use of a simple Goal-Plan-Do-Review problem-solving sequence. Although this may start out as an entirely external strategy, it may become internalized with practice.

Self-Talk Procedures

Another relatively simple self-instructional procedure involves teaching the patient to "talk themselves through" tasks. (Cicerone and Wood, 1987; Cicerone and Giacino, 1992). This serves to prevent unwanted behaviors, while simultaneously encouraging planning and self-monitoring and attentional focus. Training begins with overt verbalization (talking out loud), then transitions to faded verbal self-instruction (whispering), and then to covert verbal mediation (inner talk). The therapeutic steps for the Self-Talk Procedure are as follows:

1) As a test of their ability, therapists can ask patients to "talk themselves through" a particular task; that is, they are asked to perform a task while talking out loud about each step of the process.

2) If this fails, as it often will, the therapist can assist the patient in breaking down a task into its component steps. This can be done either by presenting the sequence of steps to the patient or, if possible, having the patient complete a formal problem-solving worksheet for the task (e.g., Goal-Plan-Do-Review). In this way, they themselves can list the various steps involved in the process.

3) Once the list is made, the therapist removes it, and the patient is again asked to perform the task while describing each step of the sequence out loud (overt verbalization).

4) Once a patient is able to do this, he or she is asked to repeat it again, but this time by whispering each step to themselves in a barely audible way (faded verbalization).

5) Finally, once a patient is able to complete a task while whispering it, he or she is asked to do it again while talking internally (inner speech). Once this is successful, a therapist can choose another task and the process is repeated.

Sohlberg and Mateer (2001) provide a useful list of the steps involved in developing relatively simple self-instructional and metacognitive strategies:

1) Identify the tasks or problems where the executive function impairments interfere (e.g., specific vocational tasks, home management tasks). Select activities that will improve the client's daily functioning, even if training effects are hyperspecific and do not generalize beyond the training tasks.

2) Identify the nature of the executive dysfunction (e.g., impulsivity, perseverative responding, lack of planning, poor problem-solving, lack of error detection, etc.).

3) Design a self-instructional procedure or choose a metacognitive strategy that will assist with that issue.

4) Model doing the task, using each step or stage in the self-instructional procedure.

5) Have the client practice doing the task while saying the self-instructional elements aloud.

6) Provide cue cards when helpful, in order to give the client prompts to use the self-instructional strategy.

7) When the client can independently perform the task using the self-instructional procedures, have the client perform the task while whispering self-instruction. Give lots of practice.

8) Fade whispering to inner speech.

9) Decide whether self-instructional procedures can be generalized to other tasks, and if so, begin using the same procedures to provide practice on other types of tasks.

10) If generalization looks possible, have the client keep a log of times when he or she used self-instruction and/or when self-instruction might have been useful even if the client did not remember to implement it.

Metacognitive strategies may also be fairly complex, and to the extent that this is true, may be usable only by those with relatively mild to moderate impairment. Complex strategies have the advantage of providing a much wider range of therapeutic challenges and experiences for a patient and may allow for the training of a wider range of target behaviors and situations, covering a wider range of applicability, and allowing for greater generalization and transfer of training.

2.6 Formal Problem-Solving Strategies

In a fundamental way, all behavior change starts with a simple model of problem-solving to guide the process. What is the problem? What are possible solutions? How do I choose one? How should I implement it? Has it worked? What should I do if it doesn't work?

Accordingly, all formal problem-solving strategies have the same basic framework. Each proceeds through a series of basic steps toward solving a problem: (1) What is the problem? (2) Set goals; (3) Plan a solution; (4) Execute the solution; and (5) Monitor feedback and make changes, if necessary.

These steps of problem-solving were utilized in studies by Von Cramon et al., (1991); Levine et al., (2000); and Cicerone at al., (2008) and are presented in Table 2-2. These steps were also utilized in the single-case studies of Ylvisaker and Feeney (1998) and Dawson et al., (2009) using a Goal-Plan-Do-Review strategy.

Table 2-2 General Framework for Rehabilitation of Executive Deficits: Problem-solving

Intervention (Reference)	Social Problem-solving Von Cramen, Von Cramon & Mai (1991)	Goal Management Training (Stop – Think – Plan) (Levine et al., 2000)	ICRP Activity Analysis (Cicerone et al., 2008)
Awareness	Problem orientation Problem definition and formulation	*Stop* Raise awareness of your own problem-solving and attention.	"What is the task that I want to accomplish?"
Anticipate / Plan	Generation of alternatives	*Define the problem* *List the steps* Take control by taking time to stop and think. State the goal: "What am I doing?"	"What are the essential parts of the task or activity?" "What abilities and skills are most likely to influence performance?" "What about the situation is likely to influence performance?" "How likely am I to be successful?"
Execute / Self-Monitor	Decision making Solution implementation	*Learn the steps* Learn strategies to help with planning and remembering to do things. Monitor task performance: "What am I doing?" Reduce anxiety and pressure and increase confidence.	Identify strategies for use during task performance Perform task Self-monitor cognitive limitations and emotional reactions Self-monitor strategy application
Self-Evaluate	Solution verification	*Check* "What is my main goal?" "Is this going to help?"	Self-evaluation Peer feedback Therapist feedback Modify goals

In the context of cognitive rehabilitation for executive dysfunction, patients are taught to gain control over their cognitive processing by learning and following a formal problem-solving strategy and implementing the solutions chosen, e.g., slowing down, avoiding impulsive responses, reflecting on one's situation, choosing among alternatives, following through with choices, keeping the goal in mind, etc..

In accordance with the BI-ISIG recommendations, patients are trained to apply the same general strategy to each new problem that they face. Initially they are taught to complete a written, structured worksheet which outlines the steps involved in the problem-solving sequence. They record the goal and the planned solution to the particular problem at hand. Then, they implement the plan and record the outcome, including both successes and failures encountered. Through frequent repetition of this same problem-solving procedure across a range of tasks, patients can learn to apply it more effectively and quickly.

The long-term goal of problem-solving training is to enable the patient to become familiar and skilled with an effective sequence for problem-solving that can be generalized to various situations with minimal use of external cues. In effect, through practice and repetition it becomes an internalized strategy with which patients can instruct themselves through internal self-talk. When internalization is not possible, an approach that utilizes an external cueing system (e.g., prompts for each step of the procedure) becomes necessary.

Formal problem-solving strategies can vary from four to 15 steps. Ylvisaker and Feeney (1998) provided a clinically useful model and procedures for problem-solving. It should be noted, however, that this model, and the steps by Ylvisaker and Feeney (1998), were excluded from the Cicerone et al., (2003) review because it was based on clinical case descriptions. Nonetheless, it is included in this manual as a useful model for clinical application of the problem-solving interventions described in Table 2-2. Table 2-3 provides a comprehensive listing of the four basic steps and the more detailed sub-steps, from Ylvisaker and Feeney (1998).

Table 2-3   Steps in Problem-solving from Ylsivaker and Feeny (1998)

Awareness	1. Recognize the existence of a problem to be solved.
	2. Indicate a personal goal that the problem is related to:
	  • "Why is this problem important and worth spending time on?"
	3. Analyze and define the main problem.
	  • Formulate questions about the problem.
	  • Analyze and record the main aspects of the problem.
	  • Distinguish between relevant and irrelevant details.

Anticipate/Plan	4. Identify information that needs to be gathered before choosing a solution. 5. Generate a list of possible solutions. • Brainstorm, thinking of as many alternatives as possible. 6. List pros and cons of each solution. 7. Choose the best option. 8. List the various steps involved in the solution chosen. 9. Learn the steps of the chosen solution.

Execute/Self-Monitor	10. Execute the solution without getting lost or stuck on one step.
	  • Avoid going off on tangents.
	  • Avoid perseveration and cognitive inflexibility.
	  • Keep in mind the goal: "Is this getting me closer to where I want to go?"

Self-Evaluate	11. Verify the effectiveness of the solution.
	  • Recognize faulty paths.
	  • Self-correct errors.
	  • Ask for feedback.

2.6.a Stages in the Training of Formal Problem-Solving Procedures

Training in the use of external problem-solving strategies will take place in three phases: acquisition; application; and adaptation. In this discussion, the basic problem-solving steps will be the Goal-Plan-Do-Review sequence taken from Ylvisaker and Feeney (1998). However, it should be noted that any series of steps that reflect the sequence validated by evidence-based research (i.e., Awareness, Plan, Execute, Self-Evaluate) can be used.

Acquisition

In the acquisition stage, the patient learns the rationale and procedures of the particular problem-solving model to be used in treatment, along with any relevant supporting materials. Successful completion of this phase occurs when the patient can recite the steps in the problem-solving model and explain the reason why each is important. He or she may be able to proceed to the application stage and be successful despite unsuccessful completion of the acquisition phase. In these cases, strategy use resembles procedural learning in which an external aid (e.g., notebook) can trigger the proper response despite the patient's inability to describe what he/she is doing.

Application

In the application phase, the patient begins to use the problem-solving model on various tasks in the clinic. The therapist will choose tasks, preferably in collaboration with the patient, that are relevant to the patient's life and that reflect an underlying deficit that interferes with his/her daily functioning. Some may be real-life tasks and some may be simulated. Using personally relevant tasks can help to facilitate generalization of the strategy being learned to tasks in "real life."

For each model of problem-solving training used with individual patients, there are forms that will help to guide their efforts. Patients will complete a new form for each new task. Therapists may initially want to model the procedures that are to be implemented to promote errorless learning. As patients carry out the designated task, it may be helpful to have them do so while saying the steps aloud.

Adaptation

In the adaptation phase, the patient applies the skills learned in the first two stages to problems and tasks outside of the clinic. This should be recorded by the participant in homework assignments, allowing the therapist to refine strategy use and monitor progress.

2.6.b Applying the Strategy to Specific Tasks

When using a formal problem-solving procedure to address a specific task, it is often helpful to have patients start with printed forms or templates that outline the major steps in the chosen problem-solving model. There are two different worksheets for the Goal-Plan-Do-Review (GDPR) procedure (Ylsivaker and Feeney, 1998). The Worksheet Form: Goal-Plan-Do-Review Model provided below is a more comprehensive worksheet that provides more structure, but is also more complex. It includes a section requiring that the patient also predict how they will do when performing the task. This worksheet also elicits more evaluation and feedback, not only from the patient, but from others as well. The patient typically will write down all relevant information pertinent to each step of the process. The use of these forms provides structure and memory triggers, which can circumvent deficits not only in executive functioning but also in memory. In this way, patients can remember the steps in any problem-solving process as they address the task. The patient should use a separate template or form for each new task.

Worksheet Form: Goal-Plan-Do-Review Model

GOAL:

What do I want to accomplish?

PLAN:

How am I going to accomplish my goal?

MATERIALS/EQUIPMENT	STEPS/ASSIGNMENTS
1.	1.
2.	2.
3.	3.
4.	4.
5.	5.

PREDICTION:

How well will I do? How much will I get done?

_____

_____

DO:

What problems did I find?	What solutions?
1.	1.
2.	2.
3.	3.

REVIEW:

How did I do?   SELF-RATING

1   2   3   4   5   6   7   8   9   10

OTHER RATING

1   2   3   4   5   6   7   8   9   10

WHAT WORKED?   **WHAT DIDN'T WORK?**

1.	1.
2.	2.
3.	3.

WHAT WILL I TRY DIFFERENTLY NEXT TIME?

_____

_____

_____

(Reproduced from Ylvisaker and Feeney, 1998, by permission)

The following worksheet is a shorter version of the GPDR intervention. Some patients may require more structure initially, and the level of cueing provided on the former version may be more appropriate for some patients. On the other hand, some patients may find the complexity and the number of steps in the previous worksheet overwhelming, and may first need to use the short-form that follows in the beginning of therapy.

Worksheet Short-Form: Goal-Plan-Do-Review Model

GOAL:

What do I want to accomplish?   What is the goal?

_____

_____

_____

_____

PLAN:

How am I going to accomplish the goal? List all the steps.

_____

_____

_____

DO:

Execute the plan.

_____

_____

_____

REVIEW:

How did I do? What worked? What didn't?

_____

_____

_____

_____

The completed problem-solving forms should be kept in a separate and easily identifiable section of the patient's Memory Notebook for later reference. When similar or related problems arise, the patient may find that he/she has already identified a successful approach to solve the problem.

Therapist recording forms for the application and adaptation stages can be found in Appendix B. These forms provide a means for an observer to document a patient's performance of specific tasks, or the various steps of specific tasks, over a given period of time.

2.6.c General Treatment Considerations with Formal Problem-Solving

As with any therapy, the severity of patients' impairment will have a major impact on the level of cueing and assistance that they need. The goal in working with those who have executive dysfunction is to enable them to succeed while providing them with the least amount of cueing and assistance necessary. If a therapist is unsure about where to start, it might be best to start with the maximum amount of scaffolding or cueing, and remove external cues (one at a time) only after the patient is able to use the problem-solving procedure successfully with maximal cues.

Some patients with milder impairment will be able to work successfully with just the four general GPDR goal headings and will respond well to general questions. These questions might include: "What should you do first/now? What do you need to do to accomplish this step? What are the important things to look for? How are you going to do that? Is there anything that you've missed?" However, some more moderately to severely impaired individuals will need to be provided with more assistance. This may involve breaking the general goals into more specific subgoals. It may also involve providing the patient with more structured cueing. So, rather than asking only open-ended questions, it may be necessary to structure the questioning by means of a multiple-choice or simple yes/no format. For the most impaired patients, therapists may need to provide answers directly in a format similar to the errorless learning that is used in memory training with severe impairment.

2.7 Metacognitive Strategy Training for Behavioral and Emotional Dysregulation

2.7.a Treating Deficits in Awareness

For those with neurocognitive unawareness, it is generally helpful to help a patient to recognize deficits by pointing out the discrepancies between self-perception and reality. In addition, Fleming and Ownsworth (2006) recommend: (1) selecting key tasks and environments in which awareness behaviors are most important within everyday activities and roles; (2) providing clear feedback and structured opportunities to help patients evaluate their performance, discover errors, and compensate for deficits; (3) using habit formation, when necessary, through repetition and procedural or implicit learning; and (4) providing education and environmental supports.

Awareness interventions often begin with a therapist pointing out an area of behavioral concern. Usually, this reflects some area in which a patient has insufficient behavioral, emotional, and/or cognitive control. Effective treatment, particularly when self-instructional strategies are being trained, usually requires assisting the patient to develop an awareness of the underlying impairments and their negative functional consequences.

The next step in the therapeutic process of treating neurocognitive unawareness is often educational. The therapist provides a patient with information about his or her condition either by informal discussion or by formal materials including handouts, leaflets, films, etc. These can provide concrete information in a simplified form to minimize demands on memory or organizational abilities. Psychoeducation about brain injury and the kinds of difficulties commonly experienced by survivors is often helpful. In describing brain injury-related impairments, it can be useful to describe symptom indicators (e.g., misplacing the car keys, forgetting people's names) rather than symptoms (e.g., memory impairment). Some individuals are not able to acknowledge broad areas of impairments, but may identify with specific symptom indicators (e.g., "I don't have a memory problem, but I have been noticing that when I get to the store, I often forget what I came for). Identifying and keeping track of symptom indicators can help an individual to gain awareness of injury-related impairments.

If a patient remains unaware of an impairment even after being provided with education and feedback, it may be necessary to identify evidence that the impairment does or does not exist. A collaborative, collegial effort can be initiated when the therapist poses a non-confrontational question: e.g., "I wonder if your difficulty reading the newspaper is related to a change in your visual attention since the accident, or if it's related to other things. Let's explore it together and see if we can gather the information we need to help improve your reading."

Toward this end, the therapist and the patient can agree to explore the evidence together. "Evidence" might include a number of observations: people not behaving as expected; conflicts between two different goals; the presence of poorly controlled negative emotions; repeated failures; repeated conflicts with others; social isolation when others stay away; and feedback from trusted significant others. Signs of impairment may also include discrepancies between a patient's past and current performance: e.g., "I used to be able to complete the crossword puzzles... remember people's birthdays... and now I can't." Engaging in a collaborative effort to identify underlying causes for these observed changes (e.g., "My memory isn't as good as it once was.") can facilitate awareness.

Individuals may provide alternative explanations for the problems they observe (e.g., "I'm not interested in the newspaper, which is why I do not remember what I read."), but supportive questioning and guided information seeking during therapy can serve to correct inaccuracies or distortions in their explanations and point toward more accurate alternatives. Together, a therapist and patient can explore potential areas of trouble and the type of neurobehavioral difficulty that may underlie it, e.g., impulsivity, inattention, hyperverbosity, or perseveration.

For patients with memory impairments and/or executive dysfunction, it can also be helpful to monitor and record systematically the rate or frequency of a patient's mistakes or problematic behavior, e.g., the number of times grocery items are not purchased when the patient refuses to use a grocery list as compared to when a grocery list is used (Alderman, et al., 1995). This can be done by the patient, by the therapist, or by trusted others. Recording difficulties and successes can provide the patient with an opportunity to compare multiple sets of observations, and identify discrepancies in order to increase knowledge about injury-related deficits and how they can be ameliorated. The goal is not to highlight a person's failures, but rather to raise awareness. Keeping track of mistakes and successes can help the patient and therapist to identify residual strengths, and to demonstrate that by capitalizing on these strengths and using compensatory strategies, the person can be more successful.

2.7.b Predict-Perform Procedure

A variant of this approach is the predict-perform technique in which a patient is asked to predict his or her performance before undertaking a task (e.g., predicted number of errors, accuracy, speed to completion, or some other aspect of success or failure) and then compare it to the actual scores obtained when the task is completed (Cheng & Man, 2006; Goverover et al., 2007; Schlund, 1999). The therapeutic steps for completing the predict-perform technique are as follows (Adapted from: Goverover, Johnston, Toglia, and Deluca, 2007):

1) Therapist introduces a task. The task can be purely paper and pencil or it can be a real or simulated IADL, e.g., prepare lunch box, pay phone bill, set up doctor appointment, organize medications, etc.

2) Patients are asked to:
   a. Define their task performance goals (e.g., two types of food will be chosen out of four, and placed into the lunch box; task completion will take 35 minutes).
   b. Predict task performance (e.g., "What do you expect the outcome will be?")
   c. Anticipate and pre-plan for any types of errors or obstacles he/she expects to encounter during the task performance (e.g., "Will this task require physical assistance; reminders, etc.?")
   d. Choose a strategy to circumvent such difficulties (e.g., written instructions, check list)
   e. Assess the amount of assistance he/she will need to successfully perform the task.

3) Following these preliminary predictions and assessments, the patient performs the task.

4) Following task completion, patients self-estimate their performance on the task (e.g., task difficulty, time required for completion, etc.). They are also asked to complete a structured self-evaluation of the task they have just performed.

5) A discussion between the therapist and patient follows, during which the patient describes his/her answers to the different questions asked and the therapist describes his/her observations to the same questions.

6) After this, patients may be encouraged to record their experience in performing the task, including tips or strategies to be successful next time.

The therapist and the patient can use the predict-perform technique to assist in identifying both behavioral and emotional factors that influence cognitive performance. Neurobehavioral problems, such as disinhibition or impulsivity, will lead the patient to not consider all of the factors that may influence their ability to perform the target tasks. The predict-perform technique can also be used to assist the patient in identifying their emotional reactions to challenging situations. A patient can rate the predicted intensity of his anger when dealing with certain situations, e.g., marital conflict, versus the actual perceived intensity of anger during the situation. Record-keeping, whether in the form of written predictions and performance ratings, or formal videotaping of a patient's behavior, can be an extremely powerful aid in helping to increase self-awareness.

In a group therapy setting, the opportunity to receive direct feedback from other patients can also be of important therapeutic value in promoting awareness. Patients will often accept and benefit from feedback about their impairments from other people with brain injuries more easily than they will accept this feedback from therapists. The importance of trust and collaboration in awareness-raising interventions cannot be overstated. The therapist must be vigilant of the patient's reactions throughout the process, recognizing that by drawing attention to impairments or difficulties, the patient could inadvertently be make to feel "stupid," embarrassed, or ashamed. Some ways a therapist can minimize negative reactions might include emphasizing a teamwork approach (e.g., "Let's work together to see if we can figure out what's getting in your way when you do the grocery shopping"), validating the patient's hard work, and instilling hope.

2.7.c Summary of Awareness Interventions Matched with Causes of Unawareness

Impairments of awareness present important challenges, practically and emotionally, to the patient, the therapist and the family. Fleming and Ownsworth (2006) have developed a very useful summary of interventions for problems with awareness, as follows:

Neurocognitive Causes

Factors Contributing to Awareness Deficits

1) Damage to the right hemisphere or parietal regions (domain specific unawareness), frontal systems or diffuse brain injury (global awareness deficits).

2) Impaired executive functioning or significant cognitive impairment contributing to the onset or maintenance or awareness deficits.

Treatment Guidelines and Interventions

1) Build a therapeutic alliance with the individual and validate any frustration or distress.

2) Select key tasks and environments in which awareness behaviors are most important within everyday activities and roles.

3) Provide clear feedback and structured opportunities to help people to evaluate their performance, discover errors, and compensate for deficits.

4) Focus on habit formation through repetition and procedural or implicit learning. Train for generalization, but be realistic and understand patients' limitations in this area.

5) Group therapy, family education and environmental supports to provide external compensation.

Psychological Causes

Factors Contributing to Awareness Deficits

Information about self is partially or fully recognized but may not be disclosed due to premorbid personality traits or coping methods. Patient may not be emotionally prepared to acknowledge their deficits.

Treatment Guidelines and Interventions

1) Build a trusting relationship with the individual and validate any frustration or distress.

2) Commence with nonconfrontational approaches to teach adaptive coping strategies (e.g., relaxation techniques) before attempting to change any maladaptive strategies that may be protecting them from emotional distress.

3) Enhance perceived control over the therapy process by presenting choices and allowing the individual to direct access.

4) Psychotherapy and adjustment counseling techniques can help to re-establish sense of self and self-mastery by exploring the subjective meaning of loss and to acknowledge grief. Grief techniques include reading books, watching movies or videos, writing personal story or poem, artwork, compiling photo album or scrap book, keeping a journal, joining a support group, etc.

5) Promote and reinforce acceptance of change, and gradually develop modified goals for the future.

Socio-Environmental Causes

Factors Contributing to Awareness Deficits

1) Information about the self is not disclosed due to concerns about how such information will be used.

2) Individuals have not had relevant information or meaningful opportunities to observe post-injury changes.

3) Cultural values impact upon the individual's understanding of the assessment or rehabilitation process.

Treatment Guidelines and Interventions

1) Clarify the rationale for the assessment or rehabilitation program, and help the person to identify any concerns (e.g., discuss the "pros and cons" of the individual being involved in an assessment to rehabilitation program).

2) Consider the timing of the intervention and need for safe and supportive opportunities to observe post-injury changes. Educate significant others to provide appropriate feedback and support. Link people to support or education groups to provide a positive social context and normalize people's experiences.

3) Seek advice from a cultural liaison officer or other professional and speak to the family and friends of the individual to develop a shared understanding.

(Reproduced in part from Fleming and Ownsworth, 2001, by permission)

2.7.d Clarifying the Nature of the Problem

Once a patient begins to accept the premise that a problem exists, the next step is to explore the nature of the problem and its various features so as to devise an effective treatment plan. To do this, information needs to be gathered from recent events or activities in which the behavior has occurred, such as encounters with family and staff. In working with a patient, these events are reviewed in order to point out potential areas of impairment: What happened during these events? What worked well? What didn't work out well? Where did things begin to go wrong?

It is helpful to use a variety of training methods to clarify and record an individual's impairments. These methods can include the use of daily logs in which patients rate or record their problems in an unstructured and open-ended fashion. In addition, it is helpful to use worksheets, which provide more structured and focused guidelines for recording relevant thoughts, feelings, and behaviors. Finally, as patients learn about themselves, they can develop personalized lists of problems and strategies. These can be collected and organized in a Memory Notebook provided for patients to retain for future use (Rath, et al., 2003).

All of these approaches serve to clarify the nature and features of the problem. Many people have difficulty identifying a problem. For example, a patient might name the problem as "I missed the bus," or "I was late to an appointment," or "My dentist was mad," and have difficulty recognizing the underlying problem is: "I have difficulty planning and monitoring my time in the morning." Having a sense of underlying/ overarching problems, in addition to defining a specific problem very concisely, is essential for formulating a solution (i.e., Which problem are we trying to solve?). Thus, if a patient has some recognition that he has a problem maintaining control over his anger, the structured worksheets can serve to clarify the nature of the problem, i.e., what were the thoughts, feelings, and actions that led up to the angry outburst? What were they thinking during the outburst? Labeling aspects of the problem in this way can be quite helpful, not only in understanding the behavior, but also in laying a foundation for regaining control over the behavior.

2.7.e Planning a Solution

Once a patient is aware that a problem exists and understands its features, the therapist can begin to help formulate a solution, which should derive directly from the nature of the problem. The solution can and often does include cognitive, behavioral, emotional, and sometimes physiological factors.

The first step in this process is for the patient to learn and remember a name or phrase for those aspects of the problem that are most obvious. Each name or phrase represents a cluster of features involved in the problem. A (nonpejorative) name can assist the patient in recognizing the nature of the problem in multiple situations, and can assist the other staff treating the patient in identifying which problem and which strategies are used to address that problem. A name or phrase should, of course, be personalized and comfortable for the patient. Ideally, the therapist facilitates the patient thinking of their own name or phrase for the problem. A sample list of selected impairments in executive functioning, their functional effects on communication (adapted from Sohlberg and Mateer, 2001) and examples of labels can be found below.

Table 2-4 Identifying and Naming Dysexecutive Disorders

DOMAIN OF IMPAIRMENT	DYSEXECUTIVE SYNDROME IN COMMUNICATION DISORDERS	POSSIBLE "NAME" OR LABEL
Initiation and Drive	Difficulty starting a behavior. Does not initiate conversation; exhibits flat affect with limited expression.	"I need to get going/get involved."
Response Inhibition	Difficulty stopping behavior. Makes inappropriate comments. Does not wait for turn in conversation.	"I need to slow down/use my brakes."
Task Impersistence	Difficulty maintaining goal-directed behavior. Looses interest in conversation. Cannot maintain a topic.	"What was my goal?"
Organization	Difficulty with sequencing and timing behavior. Poor verbal organization. Jumps from topic to topic. Seems to talk "around a subject" and not get to the main idea.	"I need to stay focused."

Reproduced in part from Sohlberg and Mateer, 2001, by permission

The process of labeling the problem enables the patient to readily identify different manifestations of a given underlying problem across a variety of situations and contexts, to step back from it, and to implement a solution that has been successful in the past. So, in the example of making inappropriate comments, the solution lies in enabling the patient to label the behavior and implement a solution. An example of labeling the problem might be: "When I'm in a large group I can get excited, and I sometimes speak without thinking." A solution might be: "I need to try to slow down. Before I say something, I need to stop, ask myself 'Does this fit?'" Patients usually require cueing initially to use the name or phrase, and the frequency on the need for cueing and the type of cue should be tracked as a measure of progress using the form provided in Appendix B.2 Adaptation Record: Multiple Tasks.

Although the process of training can vary from patient to patient, it is often helpful to approach the problem systematically with a structured problem-solving sequence (e.g., Goal-Plan-Do-Review). First, a list of all possible solutions is developed, with minimal effort to censor or inhibit the choices. While this approach may seem counter-intuitive, this approach provides the opportunity for the patient to engage in the task as well as to practice and learn self-management strategies for neurobehavioral problems. Then, the pros and cons of each possibility can be more directly examined. One way of considering the pros and cons for each potential solution might include making a list of possible unintended consequences. For each solution that the patient generates an unintended consequence, the patient can be taught a strategy through which they can eventually produce a more appropriate response (Rath et al., 2006).

As noted above, the goal of metacognitive strategy training is to remove obstacles to self-regulation and problem-solving. Collaboration with a psychologist is sometimes necessary to address the emotional reactions and negative self-statements characteristic of patients who are recovering from a brain injury. Statements or beliefs like "I'm stupid," or "I'm never going to learn this," trigger emotional reactions that interfere with problem-solving. The focus of therapy may be on decreasing impulsivity, slowing down, and thinking before acting, as these things influence problem-solving or planning. Therapy may need to simultaneously focus on removing negative self-talk in the form of cognitive distortions and irrational thoughts with the assistance of psychotherapy. For both the cognitive and emotional components of executive functioning, the patient should be encouraged to use self-talk to place the situation in objective perspective to enhance self-control. It sometimes helps to use the idea of turning to a "coach in your head" to obtain advice (Ylvisaker & Feeney, 1998). Additionally, some patients experience physiological responses to these negative self-attributions or beliefs that can include increased rate of respiration, sweating, and a subjective sense of anxiety and panic. Relaxation training, including breathing exercises, guided imagery or thought stopping provided by a psychologist, can be an important component of therapy.

2.7.f Executing, Monitoring, and Adapting

Next, the patient and therapist collaboratively choose one solution, and the patient can begin to try it out, first by means of role play and then in vivo, implementing the strategy in the problematic situation.

At this stage of therapy, it is very important for the patient to monitor his/her behavior as they try new strategies to function in real-world practical situations. For example, if the focus of therapy is to assist the patient in the self-regulation of anger and how anger influences their social behavior or problem-solving activities of daily living (e.g., solving a financial problem with your spouse), providing the patient with tools to assist with self-monitoring of affect can assist with problem-solving. Some patients may benefit from using a 10-point scale in which 0 is "no anger at all," and 10 is "the most intense you have ever experienced," to determine at what level does anger begin to become a problem or interfere with the task at hand? Teaching the patient to ask questions like, "What do you think, or feel, or do, when that happens? What should you do before it gets to the danger zone?" In these situations, it helps to separate their emotional response to the situation from the cognitive strategies they need to solve the functional problem at hand. Over time and with practice, patients may be able to avoid automatic emotional reactions in favor of more thoughtful, deliberate responses, e.g., calmly looking at one's thoughts, accepting feelings, slowing down, responding more appropriately, engaging in breathing exercises or relaxation exercises when needed, listening to music, or taking a break.

2.8 Complex Evidence-Based Programs for the Rehabilitation of Impairments of Executive Functions

2.8.a Problem-Solving Group Protocol: Rusk Institute

Researchers at the Rusk Institute of Rehabilitation Medicine have developed a 24-session treatment manual to teach individuals with acquired brain damage to problem-solve more effectively (Langenbahn, Rath, Hradil, Litke, Tucker & Diller L., 2008; Sherr, et al., Unpublished Manucript). These 24 sessions are grouped into two sets of 12 sessions each. The first set consists of 12, two-hour group sessions that address self-regulation problems and aspects of motivation. These sessions are designed to: (1) increase patients' awareness of the deleterious effects of poor emotional self-regulation on their cognitive functioning; and (2) develop ways of managing the intrusion of uncontrolled affect into the thinking process.

The second set of 12, two-hour sessions is designed to increase awareness of barriers to "clear thinking" caused by injury-related impairments. The last few sessions of the protocol integrate the two separate sections (emotional self-regulation and clear thinking), and emphasize the need to address both together.

Behavioral self-regulation and cognitive problem-solving (i.e., clear thinking) are equally important to a successful outcome, particularly in real-world stressful situations. In order to solve problems in a cognitively effective manner, individuals have to be able to control those emotional reactions that interfere with their ability to think clearly and effectively. These reactions are often associated with "negative self-talk" in the form of cognitive distortions or misattributions. Examples include: "I have to do a perfect job;" or "I'm a failure;" or "I have to be in complete control or it will be a disaster." In treating this negative self-talk, it is typically necessary to help patients recognize and label their distortions before they can begin to counteract and change them.

Throughout the course of the program, patients are provided with a variety of training materials including a daily log, worksheets, and a personal strategy list. Participants are expected to complete weekly homework assignments. They are also provided with a "Self-Regulation Worksheet" which they can use to record their thoughts, feelings and actions. This serves as an opportunity for self-reflection and analysis of their problems with behavioral dysregulation. It also offers systematic guidelines for evaluating outcomes and making modifications to their strategies to improve results.

A variety of treatment techniques are employed to assist with the training. These include modeling, role-play, and "consolidation sessions" in which group leaders meet with members for one hour once a week to review the group materials and to cue members to think about what they have learned. Modeling and role-play techniques, in particular, are employed to promote internalization of both self-regulation strategy use and self-questioning.

In an evaluation of the program, Rath et al. (2003) found that participants improved in problem-solving, particularly with regard to executive functioning, problem-solving self appraisal, and self-appraised emotional self-regulation and clear thinking; they also noted improvements in objective observer ratings of role-played scenarios.

It should be noted that the program presupposes that the leaders of the group are competent in neuropsychological rehabilitation, including group therapy. It also presupposes that patients have relatively mild cognitive deficits only, and are capable of sustaining attention for two-hour periods, taking notes, giving and receiving feedback, objectively stating their strengths and weaknesses, and relating to others with appropriate social skills.

Because the program requires a level of cognitive ability that goes far beyond that needed for the basic formal problem-solving approach described above, it may not be appropriate for patients with moderate to severe impairment. Moreover, the Rusk program was developed specifically for use in a group format, and its use in an individual treatment modality has not been validated. However, work is underway to develop a variant of the program for use as individual treatment with patients who have severe impairment (Langenbahn et al., 2008; Sherr et al., 2008).

Problem-Solving Group Protocol: Worksheets

Two worksheets are used, one for self-regulation and one for clear thinking. They are used to train members to be aware of the problems, to internalize a system to analyze their responses to problems, and to develop better ways of dealing with them. The problems analyzed are those that are reported in members' logs, or those reported by past group members. A summary of these worksheets is provided below and the complete materials can be found at: http://rusk.med.nyu.edu/professionals/continuing-education.

Emotional Regulation Worksheet

Observe Present

Patient mentally replays an event so that it can be analyzed; then identifies the immediate trigger of an emotional response as well as the physical sensations, behaviors, thoughts, assumptions and emotions associated with it.

Analyze Past

Patient traces back an event to its precursors and remote triggers, then identifies the precipitating context of the event and the warning signs of loss of emotional control and self-regulation.

Plan for Future

Patient examines the success or failure of the strategies that were used and proposes new strategies that could be used in the future.

Clear Thinking Worksheet

Observe Present

Patient analyzes a problematic situation that occurred in their lives (e.g., an example from their log) or one provided by other group members. Patient is asked to provide an initial definition of the problem, goals for desired outcome, action taken, positive vs. negative consequences of the action.

Analyze Past

This section contains a brief review of the self-regulation worksheet; the repetition is to encourage the consistent use of self-regulation techniques.

Plan for Future

Patients are encouraged to broaden their initial view of the problem. Members are asked to revise via self-questioning the initial statement of the problem definition, the goals for desired outcome, the perceived behavioral options, the evaluation of alternate solutions, and the follow through after the problem is solved.

A copy of the Rusk Problem-Solving Protocol by Sherr, Langenbahn, Simon, Rath, and Diller (Unpublished Manuscript) can be found at: http://rusk.med.nyu.edu/professionals/continuing-education.

2.8.b Anger Management Therapy Programme: Royal Rehabilitation Centre

The Anger Management Therapy Programme is a five- to eight-week, individual therapy program (Medd & Tate, 2000), based on Novaco's (1975) model of anger management, but modified for acquired brain injury. According to this model, based on cognitive behavioral principles, anger is a manifestation of arousal and the cognitive labeling of arousal. Treatment involves the use of metacognitive strategies by which patients are taught to control their anger, in part, by modifying the underlying thoughts and labels that reinforce it.

The program is structured into three stages. In the first, the focus is on psychoeducation about the principles of brain injury and how subsequent anger management problems can arise. This includes a simple model of anger, demonstrating how events can trigger angry episodes. In the second stage, interventions are designed to increase participants' awareness of their own anger by probing for cognitive, physical, and emotional changes that occur when anger is aroused. In the third stage, interventions focus on learning and using strategies to more effectively manage angry responses. These strategies include relaxation, self-talk, challenging cognitions, assertiveness training, distraction, and time-outs. The reader is encouraged to review the references above for a detailed explanation of this intervention.

2.9 Strategic and Tactical Goal Writing in the Rehabilitation of Impairment of Executive Functions

PATIENT UK: Goals for the use of Goal Management Training

Long-Term Strategic Goal

Mr. UK will apply problem-solving strategies with visual support in daily living functional activities at home and in the community in 90% of opportunities.

Monthly Strategic Treatment Goal for Training in Executive Functioning

Possible Strategic Goal #1: Initiate/Continue _____ stage (e.g., acquisition, application, adaptation) of formal problem-solving strategy training in executive protocol.

Possible Strategic Goal #2: Initiate/Continue _____ stage (e.g., acquisition, application, adaptation) of metacognitive strategy training for problem solving in executive protocol.

Possible Strategic Goal #3: Initiate/Continue executive function protocol for behavioral dysregulation.

Short-Term Tactical Treatment Goals

STGa: Mr. UK will state all steps to address a given problem in a structured clinical setting with 100% accuracy across two sessions.

STGb: Mr. UK will independently generate a list of possible solutions, given a problem scenario in a structured setting with 90% accuracy across two sessions.

STGc: Mr. UK will independently apply a chosen solution which best solves a given problem in a structured setting with 90% accuracy across two sessions.

STGd: Mr. UK independently review the outcome of the chosen solution in a structured setting in 90% opportunities across two sessions.

STGe: Mr. UK will independently demonstrate evidence of the use of problem solving strategies in an unstructured situation by completion of the problem solving template twice weekly across one month.

PATIENT SR: Goals for use of Predict-Perform-Evaluate

Long-Term Strategic Goal

Ms. SR will demonstrate ability to adequately predict objective performance on completion of actual academic tasks to increase independence with required return to school activities.

Monthly Strategic Treatment Goal for Training in Executive Functioning

Possible Strategic Goal #1: Initiate/Continue _____ stage (e.g., acquisition, application, adaptation) of formal problem solving strategy training in executive protocol.

Possible Strategic Goal #2: Initiate/Continue _____ stage (e.g., acquisition, application, adaptation) of metacognitive strategy training for problem-solving in executive protocol.

Possible Strategic Goal #3: Initiate/Continue executive function protocol for behavioral dysregulation.

Short-Term Tactical Treatment Goals:

STGa: Ms. SR will independently predict time and accuracy of performance on trials of academic tasks within 10% of actual performance in 90% of opportunities.

STGb: Ms. SR will independently generate strategies to improve ability to complete tasks with enhanced accuracy and time, based on review of objective previous performance on trials of academic tasks.

STGc: Ms. SR will independently predict adequate time to complete assignments by making entries in academic planner in 90% of opportunities across one month.

PATIENT KB: Goals for use of Video Review/Self-evaluation

Long-Term Strategic Goal

Mr. KB will identify inappropriate pragmatic skills in social and work-related scenarios while reviewing a video-recorded role-play clinical interaction in 90% of opportunities.

Monthly Strategic Treatment Goal for Training in Executive Functioning

Possible Strategic Goal #1: Initiate/Continue _____ stage (e.g., acquisition, application, adaptation) of formal problem solving strategy training in executive protocol.

Possible Strategic Goal #2: Initiate/Continue _____ stage (e.g., acquisition, application, adaptation) of metacognitive strategy training for problem solving in executive protocol.

Possible Strategic Goal #3: Initiate/Continue executive function protocol for behavioral dysregulation.

Short-Term Tactical Treatment Goals:

STGa: Mr. KB will identify when he does not follow directions in 90% of opportunities.

STGb: Mr. KB will identify when does not respond appropriately to conflicting situations in 90% of opportunities.

STGc: Mr. KB will identify when he does not stay on topic in discourse in 90% of instances.

STGd: Mr. KB will identify when he does not use appropriate topic choice in discourse in 90% of instances.

STGe: Mr. KB will identify when he does not use appropriate turn taking skills in conversation in 90% of instances.

3. Rehabilitation for Impairments of Memory

3.1 Introduction

Deficits in memory functioning are common in individuals following acquired neurological damage and can have a significant impact on functional independence. Memory itself is a complex set of skills, comprising a number of subprocesses: (1) attention; (2) encoding; (3) storage; and (4) retrieval (Sohlberg & Mateer, 2001).

At its most basic level, attention involves simple alertness and arousal. At higher levels, it involves working memory, sustained concentration, vigilance, and divided attention. Attention is often considered a necessary prerequisite to memory. If an individual is unable to pay attention, new information will not "get in" or be encoded, and he or she will be unable to remember this information later. For this reason, individuals with attentional impairments may report that they have memory problems because the experience of not remembering things may cause more salient functional impairment.

Information that a person is able to attend to remains in the short-term memory for just a few seconds, and can be encoded and stored in long-term memory. Encoding refers to the ability to assign meaningfulness to verbal or nonverbal sensory information so that it can be recalled later. Storage refers to the transfer of information into long-term memory which is a permanent memory store, sometimes referred to as retention. Once information is stored in long-term memory it can be retrieved. Retrieval refers to the search for, or activation of, existing memory traces. Retrieval problems are known to be related to faulty organization of information at the time of encoding.

There are several types of long-term memory. Most generally, long-term memory can be divided into declarative and procedural memories. Declarative memory, also called explicit memory, is purposefully learned, stored, and retrieved. Examples of declarative memories include remembering a friend's birthday, or the name of the country's first president. On the other hand, procedural memory does not rely on conscious recall, but rather on "accidental" or implicit learning. Procedural memory is often involved in learning motor skills. Evidence for the distinction between declarative and procedural memories comes from individuals with hippocampal lesions. These individuals are able to benefit from implicit learning and perform better with repetition on a motor task (i.e., pegboard assembly task) despite the fact that the person may have no explicit memory of having ever before completed the task.

It is sometimes useful to further specify types of declarative memory. For example, semantic memory includes memories of facts and abstract concepts (i.e., definitions of words). Episodic memory includes context-specific memories of things that happen (i.e., remembering where you where upon learning that Kennedy was shot). A further subdivision of episodic memory is autobiographical memory, which refers to memories for personally-relevant events.

A final way of distinguishing memory types has to do with the temporal relation to the information being remembered. Retrospective memory includes all memories for information that has already occurred, while prospective memory includes memory for events that will happen in the future (i.e., I have a doctor's appointment next Tuesday), and requires an individual to remember to remember.

3.2 Impairments of Memory Deficits and Brain Injury

Memory functions rely on complex pathways and interconnections between brain regions, and are not usually localized to specific brain regions. Therefore, damage to any part of a pathway that is necessary for a particular memory function can cause impairment.

However, there are some general brain regions that have been shown to play particularly central roles in memory. It is believed that the frontal lobes and subcortical processes are the primary brain structures involved in the retrieval of information. Individuals with frontal lobe damage are often unsuccessful in attempts to freely recall information, but they may be able to retrieve this information when provided with cues. Damage to subcortical areas such as the hippocampus, amygdala, or striatum can disrupt declarative memory for facts and events. Damage to the cerebellum and basal ganglia can disrupt procedural memory involved in motor learning, though disruptions in procedural or implicit memory are not commonly seen in individuals with traumatic brain injury.

3.3 BI-ISIG Recommendations for Memory Dysfunction

The BI-ISIG Cognitive Rehabilitation Task Force of ACRM recommends, as a Practice Standard, the use of "Memory Strategy Training" for the treatment of "mild memory impairments from traumatic brain injury, including the use of internalized strategies (e.g., visual imagery) and external memory compensations (e.g., notebooks). (Cicerone et al., 2000; Cicerone et al., 2005; & Cicerone et al., 2011).

There are a number of internal strategies that have been used successfully in the treatment of memory impairment. These include all of those techniques that come under the heading of "mnemonic" techniques. Internalized strategies tend to require relatively high-level conscious and deliberate control by those who use them and, as a result, are often more difficult than those strategies that are external. For this reason, they are most appropriate for those patients with only mild to, at worst, moderate memory impairment.

In addition, the BI-ISIG recommends external compensations, as a Practice Guideline, for those individuals with more severe memory impairments after stroke or TBI, with direct application to functional activities. The hallmark of these strategies is the use of a reference or device that is external to the patient. The general goal is to bypass impaired functions by providing an alternative strategy to record and retain information (as with a Memory Notebook) or to cue adaptive behaviors (as with an alarm system).

Included among these external compensations are various techniques designed to enhance memory organization, including written planning systems, electronic planners, computerized systems, auditory or visual systems, and task-specific aids (such as Post-it® notes, pocket notebooks, home calendars, etc.). In this regard, external Memory Notebook strategies can be quite successful (Ownsworth & McFarland, 1991).

The BI-ISIG recommends, as a Practice Option, that group based interventions may be considered for remediation of memory deficits after TBI (Cicerone et al., 2011).

For people with severe memory impairments after TBI, the BI-ISIG indicates, as a Practice Option, that errorless learning techniques may be effective for learning specific skills or knowledge, with limited transfer to novel tasks or reduction in overall functional memory problems (Cicerone et al., 2011).

3.4 A General Framework for Rehabilitation of Impairments of Memory

Treatment of memory deficits research has typically shown that, as with treatment in any area of cognitive rehabilitation, a number of factors influence outcome. These include the severity of the memory impairment, the complexity of the memory strategy chosen or tasks utilized, and the patient's level of self-awareness.

In general, persons with less severe memory impairment and minimal or no deficits in self-awareness tend to do well and may make use of various memory rehabilitation strategies, whether those strategies are internal or external.

In contrast, those patients with more severe memory deficits and/or significant problems with self-awareness tend to do better with strategies that are external rather than internal. Accordingly, internal strategies, i.e., memory mnemonics, may not be as useful for those individuals with moderate to severe impairment.

As derived from the evidence-based reviews and recommended by BI-ISIG, two overall approaches to the rehabilitation of memory disorders will be discussed:

1) external memory compensations, and

2) memory (metacognitive) strategy training.

Complex evidence-based programs for memory training will also be reviewed later in this chapter. Within these approaches are a number of more specific techniques that are described. As a general rule, tactical goals will tend to be drawn from the more specific classifications of techniques or methods. Table 3-1 provides an overview of the two approaches to memory rehabilitation and the techniques that are used to address these two approaches that will be reviewed in this chapter.

Table 3-1 Approaches and Techniques in the Rehabilitation of Memory

APPROACHES	TECHNIQUES

External Compensations	Orientation Notebook
	    Errorless Learning Technique
	    Spaced Retrieval Technique
	    Chaining Technique
	Electronic Device
	    Cell phone
	    Pager
	    Alarms
	Memory Notebook

Memory Strategy Training	Association Techniques
	    Visual — Verbal Association
	    Visual — Verbal Schematics
	    Visual Peg Method
	    Method of Loci
	Organizational and Elaboration Techniques
	    First Letter Mnemonics
	    Semantic Clustering
	    PQRST
	    Use of Humor
	    Storytelling

In the case of both internal and external strategies, the long-term goal is to enable the patient to perform real-world functionally and personally relevant tasks. No such presumption of independent use is made with the method of errorless learning, which is designed to teach specific information to patients with severe memory impairment.

Learning of the target behavior occurs through the active control and involvement of the therapist. Patients with severe persisting memory impairment, unless they happen to also have good awareness of their impairment, are generally unable to assume control and direction over their use. Even if they are successful with the acquisition of the target behavior through training using errorless learning, it is typically without their conscious control over its use or application. A decision tree outlining the general options in treatment planning of memory impairment is provided in Figure 3-1 below:

Figure 3-1   Decision Tree for Treatment Planning In Memory Dysfunction

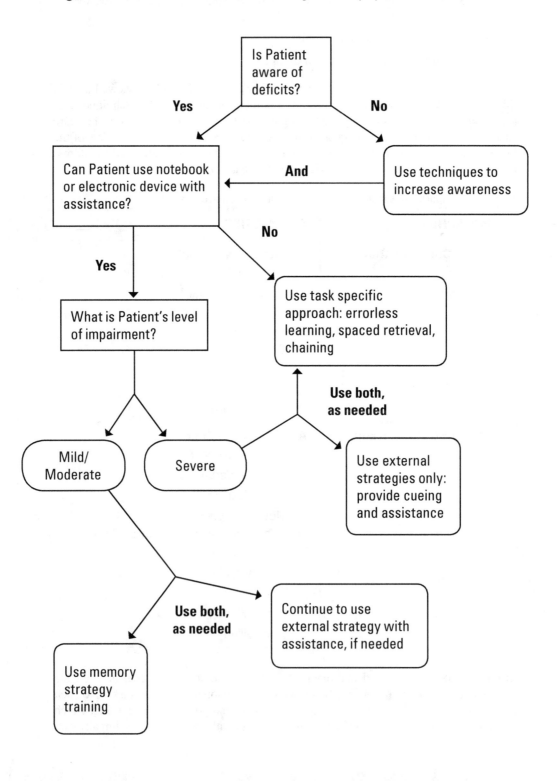

3.5 External Memory Compensations

In the rehabilitation of disorders of memory, several types of external devices have been commonly employed. These devices include: notebooks or other written planning systems; electronic planners; smart cell phones; computerized systems; auditory or visual systems; and task-specific aids.

The decision regarding which external device(s) to use in any given situation involves a number of factors, including: (1) the particular task that the patient wishes to perform; (2) the patient's goals, abilities, disabilities, and preferences; (3) the physical features (or limitations) of available technology; and (4) the environment in which technology is going to be used.

3.5.a General Guidelines for External Memory Compensations

1) To be effective, the patient must have constant and easy access to the external device or Memory Notebook, and be able to carry it with him/her at all times.

2) All staff and family members working with a patient need to be trained in the application and use of the memory system.

3) For the more severely impaired patients, success is likely to be measured by their ability to perform the procedure (procedural memory), not their ability to describe what they should do (declarative memory). In addition, the use of errorless learning and increased prompting will be necessary with the more severely impaired individual.

4) Therapists should be prepared for the fact that it takes time for patients to learn external memory strategies. Initial training is often difficult, but can be successful over time.

5) For training purposes, it is helpful to have the patient perform activities that he/she finds reinforcing, interesting and rewarding.

6) Patients need to have a minimal level of self-awareness, especially of their memory deficits. If they do not, development of personal awareness needs to be addressed (see section 2.7 Metacognitive Strategy Training for Behavioral and Emotional Dysregulation).

7) Executive functions may have a significant impact on a patient's ability to learn and implement external memory strategies. Accordingly, executive cognitive functioning needs to be evaluated and any deficits should be addressed in the context of memory treatment.

8) The goal of using external devices is to provide a means by which a patient can perform important, functional tasks in his/her daily life. Toward this end, it is often necessary for the therapist to conduct a detailed analysis of the tasks that a person needs or hopes to be able to perform.

9) Most patients need cues, especially early in treatment, but the ultimate goal is to eliminate cueing or prompting as soon as possible. In general, rapid fading of cues is more effective for patients with better memories and those learning simpler tasks. Gradual fading of cues is more effective for patients with more severe impairment and those learning more complex tasks.

3.5.b Memory Notebook Types

There are two variants of the external Memory Notebook approach, based on level of complexity and the ability and needs of the patient. Patients with very severe memory impairment and/or persisting post-traumatic amnesia can benefit from training in the utilization of an Orientation Book using several different strategies (errorless learning, spaced retrieval, and chaining). Patients with mild to moderately severe memory impairment can be trained to use a Memory Book.

Orientation Book and Strategies for Severe Memory Impairment

The Orientation Book often has two parts: a) an autobiographical orientation page; and b) additional orientation information, depending on the need of the patient. The autobiographical orientation page is a single sheet of paper, often in a plastic page protector, which the patient has available at all times. All relevant, but basic, personal information is recorded on a single sheet, preferably in front of the patient or within easy reach. This tool is primarily for patients in post-traumatic amnesia and is in a "read only" form. Initially, staff and family record pertinent and relevant information on the page and the patient is cued to refer to it to promote orientation. Prospectively and routinely orienting the patient with the Orientation Book may assist with preventing anxiety or agitation. An example of the autobiographical orientation page is as follows:

Form 3-1   Autobiographical Orientation Page

Patient Name:_____   Date:_____

My name is: _____

I am _____ years old

I was born on: _____

My phone number is: _____

Right now I am in the city of: _____

The date today is: _____

Right now I am at a: _____

I was injured on: _____

The kind of injury that I have is a: _____

(Others, as driven by the patient's questions)

Depending on the needs of the patient, the Orientation Book can be expanded to include:

- the current date
- location
- names and pictures of staff (e.g., therapists, nurses)
- injury details
- names and pictures of family, friends, or pets
- personal messages that may be helpful or appropriate, such as notes from family when they last visited.

Care should be taken to make the information as user friendly as possible with a minimum of visual clutter. As much as is possible, the patient should be trained to refer to the book, typically with cueing, to answer his/her own questions.

Errorless learning, spaced retrieval and chaining are three different methods that can be utilized to promote the acquisition of functionally important and relevant behaviors utilizing preserved procedural leaning and memory systems. These methods can be utilized for a variety of domain-specific target behaviors, such as steps in balancing a checkbook or recalling a telephone number, but also for acquisition of steps or sequences of behavior to utilize a Memory Notebook.

Errorless Learning Technique

The most common method of presenting information using an errorless learning paradigm is to simply make a statement and ask the patient to recall the statement without delay. For example:

1. My name is Dr. Smith. "What is my name?"
2. Your son lives in Evansville. "Where does your son live?"
3. Your room number is 104. "What is your room number?"

A slightly more complex method is a simple command with a conditional clause attached, indicating when the command is to be executed:

1. When you pick up the phone, say "Hello, this is Evelyn. What should you say when you pick up the phone?"
2. Before you sit down, make sure that you feel for the back of the chair. "What should you do before you sit down?"
3. When you swallow, you should tuck your chin like this (therapist demonstrates). "What should you do when you swallow?"

The errorless learning method can be used for training the patient for basic autobiographical information in the Orientation Book, as exemplified on Form 3-1.

Form 3-2 Errorless Learning Protocol for Orientation

PERSON (turn to Orientation page)

1. "Your name is _____." (pause) "What is your name?"
2. "You are _____ years old." (pause) "How old are you?"
3. "You were born _____." (pause) "When were you born?"
4. "Your phone number is _____" (pause) "What is your phone number?"

PLACE (stay on Orientation page)

1. "We are in Indianapolis." (pause) "What city are we in right now?"
2. "You are in a clinic right now." (pause) "What type of place are you in right now?"

INJURY (stay on Orientation page)

1. "The date of your injury was _____." (pause) "What was the date of your injury?"
2. "You have a _____." (pause) "What kind of injury do you have?"

CALENDAR (turn to calendar)

1. "This year is _____." (pause) "What year is it right now?"
2. "This month is _____." (pause) "What month is it right now?"

Orientation Record

In general, errorless learning is the foundation for all information to be presented to patients with severe memory impairment. The therapist should remember to provide cues freely as needed. Frequent repetition is helpful. It is also helpful to train a skill or present information in the actual setting or context in which it will be used. Do not allow guessing or trial-and-error learning. The goal is to not allow a patient to make a mistake on which the patient may perseverate repeatedly. Errorless learning can be used not only for presenting simple information, but also in conjunction with slightly more complex techniques such as spaced retrieval and chaining.

Spaced Retrieval Technique

Before beginning to use the spaced retrieval technique (Brush & Camp, 1998), it is helpful to screen a patient's ability to remember information using errorless learning. Spaced retrieval is identical to errorless learning except that the patient is asked to retain the information for progressively longer periods of time. As such, the patient may be told what the therapist's name is, and then asked to repeat that after progressively longer intervals (e.g., immediate, 15-second delay, and 30-second delay). The duration of the interval can be modified and lengthened according to patient performance. An example of a spaced retrieval training protocol follows.

Form 3-3   Spaced Retrieval Training Protocol

Patient Name:_____   Date:_____

1. Immediate

"Today we are going to practice remembering my name. My name is
_____. What is my name?"

Trial 1 _____   Trial 2 _____   Trial 3 _____   Total Correct _____

If a patient responds incorrectly at immediate recall, simply repeat the
statement. Once a patient is correct on trial 1, 2, or 3, proceed to short
delay

2. 15-Second Delay

"Good. I want to help you see if you can remember my name for a
longer period of time. Let's try again and see if you can remember
my name after 15 seconds. My name is _____." After a
15-second delay, the therapist would then ask "What is my name?"

Trial 1 _____   Trial 2 _____   Trial 3 _____   Total Correct _____

If a patient responds incorrectly at short delay, say "Actually my name
is _____." After a 15-second delay, the therapist would again ask
"What is my name?" If the patient cannot remember the therapist's
name after 15 seconds, it may be appropriate to try a 5-second or
10-second delay. Once a patient is correct on trial 1, 2, or 3 with a
15-second delay, proceed to a 30-second delay.

3. 30-Second Delay

"You are doing well remembering my name for a longer period of time
and that's the idea. I would like to see if you can always remember
my name. Let's see if you can remember my name after 30-seconds.
My name is _____." After a 30-second delay, the therapist
would then ask "What is my name?"

Trial 1 _____   Trial 2 _____   Trial 3 _____   Total Correct _____

If a patient responds incorrectly at long delay, say, as at short delay:
"Actually my name is _____. What is my name?" If the
patient completes the task successfully without making three errors at
any of the delays, spaced retrieval is appropriate.

Reproduced from Brush & Camp, 1998, by permission

The length of the intervals can be adjusted according to patient performance as well
as the complexity of information to be remembered. The information presented to be
remembered can also be accompanied by visual information that may assist in learning
and retrieval. Carefully recording and analyzing data over training trials can provide
insights into the conditions which maximize learning. Using a Record Form like the one
below can assist.

Form 3-4 Spaced Retrieval Record Form

Patient Name:_____ Date:_____

Information being presented: _____

Trial	Imm	Delay in: _____Seconds _____Minutes														
		1	2	3	4	5	6	8	10	12	16	20	24	28	32
1															
2															
3															
4															
5															
6															
7															
8															
9															
10															
11															
12															

The user can indicate if the recall was correct or incorrect for each trial by placing a (+) or (-) in box corresponding to the delay interval. Obviously, the delay interval can be modified according to the patient need.

(Reproduced from Brush & Ca mp, 1998, by permission)

Chaining Technique

Any complex task represents a sequence of specific behaviors or a chain, i.e., a chain of steps, each of which is strongly linked to the steps next to it. The completion of one step in the sequence serves as a cue for the completion of the next step. By the same token, each step serves to reinforce the one that came before it. In this way, a strong set of connections is established between adjoining steps in the sequence.

However, patients with severe memory impairment often have difficulty establishing a new chain of behavior, or sometimes even executing a chain acquired prior to brain injury. Chaining is a technique which can be used to train patients to perform sequences of steps by means of procedural memory, in which each item is learned automatically, as an isolated unit, which is then mechanically linked with the items before and after. Each step serves as a cue for the next step but, in chaining, this typically occurs without the patient recognizing that the overall sequence of steps represents anything meaningful. Rather, the task is performed automatically and reflexively, without conscious and deliberate intent.

Chaining can be used with either verbal or visual information. Often it is used with both. It is also helpful, in order to enhance memory recall, to incorporate motor movements when appropriate to the task being performed.

The use of a chaining technique typically begins with a thorough analysis in which a complex task is broken down into its various component steps, each of which needs to be clearly identified and defined. For example, in a simple face-washing task, the sequence might be broken down into: (1) splash water on my face; (2) rub soap on it; (3) splash water on it again; and (4) dry it. Having done this, the therapist can begin the process of linking each step with the next one by means of chaining.

There are two basic types of chaining: forward and backward. In forward chaining, the therapist begins with the first step in the chain and guides the patient in performing it. Once he or she is able to perform that first step, the second step is introduced and the patient is guided to perform both together. When that is successful, the third step is introduced, and the patient is again guided to perform all three together. This continues until all the steps in the sequence are complete. By this means, each step in the sequence is linked together with the one coming before it and the one coming after it.

Backward chaining is identical, with the exception that the steps are taught from the last in the sequence to the first, rather than from first to last. A form of backward chaining termed "vanishing cues" is a process for teaching new information in which prompts are provided and then gradually removed (Glisky et al., 1986).

Generally, in backward chaining, the therapist will begin by demonstrating all the steps in a complex sequence and then will gradually begin to omit more and more of the final steps in the sequence. For example, after showing a patient the entire sequence of a four-step task, the therapist will perform steps 1 through 3 and then guide the patient in performing step 4. When this is successful, the therapist will perform steps 1 and 2 and then guide the patient in performing steps 3 and 4. This will continue until the patient can perform the entire sequence.

A summary of this technique from the research literature is provided in Evans et al. (2000). They also present an example in which they taught a subject the names of people along with their photographs. The subject was presented with a photograph and directly told the name, which they immediately wrote down. Next, when shown the photograph, the subject was told and shown all the letters of the corresponding name, with the final letter omitted. The subject then provided the name. This process was repeated, with removal of the next letter from the end of the name, until the subject was shown the photograph and requested to generate the name given only the initial letter of the name. If the subject made an error, they were immediately informed that their response was inaccurate and told the correct response. They were never encouraged to guess. Conclusions of the research indicated the new learning was more successful with a process that prevented errors.

A copy of a worksheet to be used with forward or backward chaining can be found on Form 3-5.

Form 3-5 Chaining Worksheet Using Errorless Learning

Patient Name:_____ Date:_____

Task: _____

Steps involved in the task:

1) _____

2) _____

3) _____

4) _____

INSTRUCTIONS: FORWARD CHAINING (FOR A FOUR-STEP TASK)

(1) Demonstrate all steps in the task sequence and label each step as you do.

> *Say:* "When you need to (perform specified task), you should do steps ___1___, ___2___, ___3___ and ___4___."

> *Do:* Perform the task for the patient.

(2) Teach step one.

> *Say:* "When you need to (perform specified task), you should begin by ___1___. What should you do when you need to (perform specified task)?"

> *Do:* Guide patient, as needed, through performance of step one.

(3) Teach step two.

> *Say:* "After you do ___1___, you should do ___2___. What should you do after you do ___1___?"

> *Do:* Guide patient, as needed, through performance of step one and two together.

(4) Teach step three.

> *Say:* "After you do ___2___, you should do ___3___. What should you do after you do ___2___?"

> *Do:* Guide patient, as needed, through performance of step one, two and three together.

(5) Teach step four.

> *Say:* "After you do ___3___, you should do ___4___. What should you do after you do ___3___?"

> *Do:* Guide patient, as needed, through performance of step one, two, three and four together.

INSTRUCTIONS: BACKWARD CHAINING (FOR A FOUR-STEP TASK)

(1) Demonstrate all steps in the task sequence and label each step as you do.

Say: "When you need to (perform specified task), you should do steps ___1___, ___2___, ___3___ and ___4___."

Do: Perform the task for the patient.

(2) Teach step four.

Say: "When you need to (perform specified task), you should begin by doing steps ___1___, ___2___, and ___3___. After you do ___3___ you need to do ___4___. What should you do when you need to after step ___3___?"

Do: Guide patient, as needed, through performance of step four.

(3) Teach step three.

Say: "When you need to (perform specified task), you should begin by doing steps ___1___ and ___2___, After you do steps ___1___ and ___2___, you should do steps ___3___ and ___4___. What should you do after you do ___1___ and ___2___?"

Do: Guide patient, as needed, through performance of steps three and four together.

(4) Teach step two.

Say: "When you need to (perform specified task), you should begin by doing step ___1___. After you do step ___1___, you should do steps ___2___, ___3___ and ___4___. What should you do after you do ___1___?"

Do: Guide patient, as needed, through performance of steps two, three and four together.

(5) Teach step one.

Say: "When you need to (perform specified task), you should begin by doing step ___1___. What should you do first to (perform specified task)?"

Do: Guide patient, as needed, through performance of steps one, two, three and four together.

Memory Notebook

Utilization of a Memory Notebook is appropriate for patients who present with mild to moderately severe memory impairment, and the patient presents with at least recognition that their memory impairment affects day-to-day activities. Memory Notebooks can and should vary as a function of complexity, depending on the patient's need. In general, it is much better to start with a simple Memory Notebook and achieve mastery with its utilization before adding other sections. These issues are addressed more fully in subsequent sections of the present chapter.

Most Memory Books begin with three core sections (Doneghy & Williams, 1998), including:

1) Daily schedule
2) Memory log
3) Things to do

These three sections can be placed on two pages attached to a simple three-ring binder, as exemplified below in Form 3-6. It is also helpful to include a section of the Memory Notebook for either a weekly or monthly calendar on which the patient can place forthcoming appointments or events, and transfer these appointments or events to their daily schedule.

Form 3-6   Memory Notebook

Patient Name:_____   Date:_____

Page 1			Page 2	
	Schedule	**Memory Log**	**Things To Do**	**Completed**
7:30	Take Medicine			
8:15	Cognitive Group			
9:00	Independent Work			
9:45	Speech Therapy			
10:30	Physical Therapy			
11:15	Memory Group			
12:00	Lunch Take Medicine			
1:00	Physical Skills Group			
1:45	Physical Skills Group			
2:30	Occupational Therapy			
3:15				
4:00				
Evening	Have dinner and have fun!!			
8:00	Take Medicine			

(Reproduced from Doneghy & Williams, 1998, by permission)

The schedule section can be completed by staff, the patient with cueing, or by the patient independently, depending on the patient's level of independence. Even when, however, the patient requires the assistance of the staff to complete their schedule, it is recommended that the patient be actively engaged in recording this information to promote orientation, procedural learning, and patient engagement in utilizing the Memory Notebook. The Memory Log is a section in which the patient is trained to make notes about particularly important information that was relevant to that event in their schedule. Rehabilitation staff participating in the different scheduled activities should cue the patient as appropriate to make these entries. It is especially helpful for one designated therapist to consistently address the "Things To Do" section with the patient until they are independent in recording and monitoring their completion of this section, as well as to promote day-to-day carry-over of therapeutically- and functionally-relevant tasks.

3.5.c Stages of Training in the Use of Memory Notebook Procedures

Training in the use of a Memory Notebook occurs over three phases: (1) acquisition; (2) application; and (3) adaptation (Sohlberg and Mateer, 2001).

Acquisition Stage

The goal for training in the acquisition stage is for the patient to learn and remember the names, location and purpose, and use (i.e., acquire semantic knowledge) for each section of the Memory Notebook. Errorless learning and/or spaced retrieval strategies may be utilized in the acquisition phase, depending on the severity of the patient's impairment in learning and memory. An example of an errorless learning protocol for acquisition of knowledge for the sections of a Memory Notebook follows.

a. The names of the notebook's sections are the Schedule, the Memory Log, and the Things To Do. What are the names of the sections of your notebook?

b. The Schedule section of your Memory Notebook is for you to record your appointments for the day. What do you record in the Schedule section?

c. The Things To Do section of your Memory Notebook is for you to record things you need or want to do that day. What do you record in the Things To Do section?

For patients who do not require errorless learning, an example of a protocol that simply requires question and answer rehearsal follows.

a. In what section of your Memory Notebook do you plan evening activities?

b. In what section of your Memory Notebook do you record future appointments?

c. In what section of your Memory Notebook do you keep your homework or things to do?

d. In what section of your Memory Notebook do you find today's date?

e. In what section of your Memory Notebook do you find what you did yesterday?

The training may also address the patient's knowledge about how to use the Memory Notebook in context of their day-to-day activities through examples as follows:

a. You will keep the notebook _____ . (Note: Family input can also be important regarding the location of the Memory Notebook when the patient is not in a clinical environment so that they can cue the patient as necessary or access the Memory Notebook when appropriate.)

b. You should review what you have recorded in the book when _____.

c. You should write in the Memory Log when _____.

d. You should record information about appointments when _____.

e. You should look at your Calendar when _____.

f. When you finish something on the Things To Do list, you should _____.

Discontinuation Criteria

Sohlberg and Mateer (2001) have suggested that optimal performance on all questions pertinent to acquisition of knowledge about the Memory Notebook is to achieve 100% accuracy on all questions for three consecutive days. However, this level of performance may not be attainable for some patients, and ultimately the clinician should decide if enough knowledge of the use of the Memory Notebook has been acquired, such that the Memory Notebook could become a useful tool for the patient to compensate for their impairment of memory functioning. If patients are able to recognize some sections of the book, have a rudimentary understanding of what those sections involve, and can use them appropriately (making use of procedural memory ability), this may be sufficient to allow them to begin using the book in a functional way. In addition, therapists do not need to wait until a patient shows competence with all sections of the book before moving to the application phase. Rather, they can begin by using only those sections of the book for which the patient has demonstrated some basic ability.

Application Stage

In the application phase, the patient begins to use the Memory Notebook in various real life and/or role play tasks in the clinical environment. The therapist will choose tasks, in collaboration with the patient, that are relevant to his/her life and that reflect an underlying deficit that interferes with daily functioning.

The therapist should allow a few minutes during or at the end of the session for the patient to record, in the Memory Log, important information from each session. The therapist may read what is written and provide constructive feedback.

The therapist records whether the patient writes in the book during each session, and records what level of cues are needed.

Adaptation Stage

In the adaptation phase, the patient applies skills learned in the first two stages to problems and tasks outside of the clinic, in community and naturalistic settings.

There are, of course, a wide variety of tasks that can be developed at this stage. In general, any task that was previously performed as a role play in the clinic can now be performed in the community The goal of therapy at this stage is for the patient to utilize their notebook for obtaining, recording and retrieving relevant information. Examples of relevant activities are provided below.

I. **Community-based information and activities** which might be accessed through in-person, telephonic, or internet resources

A. Location of... Phone # of... Name of...

1) Local store
2) Government agency
    a. Medicaid office
    b. Medicare office
    c. Vocational Rehabilitation

3) Public sector resources
    a. Brain Injury Association
    b. Library
4) Physician's or Psychologist's office

B. Cost of…
  1) By phone call to local store
  2) By going to internet website

II. Using notebook to remember to perform a future action

A. At home exercises:
  1) Bring in the _____ item from home
  2) Tell your family member something
    a. One thing done at therapy today
    b. To call the therapist
    c. Plan a special event for your spouse

B. Record homework assignments, appointments and things to do:
  1) Homework assignments
  2) Appointments
    a. Doctor's appointment
    b. Meeting with agent/counselor
  3) Invitation to event
    a. Invitation to meeting
    b. Invitation to party

III. In session exercises (with prearranged "Things to Do" list):

A. Turn to the _____ section of the notebook and do what it says on the Post-it® note.
  1) Arithmetic computation
  2) Call the front desk, home, etc.
  3) Bring an item to someone in the clinic
  4) Add/Cancel an appointment
  5) Schedule a future event
  6) Write down the CNN sequence (see the next section) and show how to do it
    a. Check your watch for the date and time
    b. Open notebook to correct day of the week
    c. Cross off the completed task on the "Things To Do" list
    d. Make a notation on the what I did today sheet
    e. Check to see what task is next

B. Read notebook entry from:
  1) Last session
  2) What you did over the weekend
  3) Other

C. Check to see if _____ is in your Memory Notebook.

D. Using notebook to record ongoing information.
  1) Daily schedule
  2) Record summaries of activities in daily sessions
  3) Homework Assignments/Projects
  4) Activities at home

Patients should also be trained in using the notebook to remember to perform future actions (prospective memory). For those with severe problems, this may involve the use of an electronic device as a reminder to perform the task.

Cross Out, Notation, and Next Activity (CNN)

When using any Memory Notebook, the sequence of steps involved in common tasks needs to become routine and automatic. At the most basic level, patients are taught the procedure of "Cross out, Notation, and Next activity" (CNN) through practical/real life tasks or role plays. The specific sequence of steps in this procedure may vary depending on the task and the ability of the patient. However, one such procedure, involving the "Things To Do" section includes the following steps: (1) Check your watch for the date and time; (2) Open your notebook to the correct day of the week; (3) Cross off the completed task; (4) On the Memory Log sheet, make a notation about the completed task; and (5) Check to determine what the next task is (Donaghy and Williams, 1998).

In this way, the CNN procedure can assist patients in learning the mechanics of using the Memory Notebook through a series of brief tasks and basic exercises conducted in therapy sessions. In one such exercise, the therapist writes a task on a note in the "Things to Do" section of the book. The patient is then asked to turn to that section, cross off the task, make a notation of it in the Memory Log, and check to see what the next task is.

Other examples of simple exercises that patients might be given include: (1) Perform _____ arithmetic calculation on a Post-it® note that has been placed by the therapist in the _____ section of the Memory Notebook; (2) Read the last weekend's notebook entry; (3) Read the notebook entry from the last session; (4) Check to see if the _____ is in your Memory Notebook; (5) Call the front desk and say _____; and (6) Bring (object) to (person) in the clinic/office.

More functional examples of in-clinic exercises and tasks include: canceling an appointment; adding an appointment; calling someone to invite him/her to dinner; sending a reminder of a meeting by phone; or calling someone to remind him/her to bring a particular item to a meeting. In all of these exercises, the tasks can be made increasingly complex as the patient's ability allows.

Sohlberg and Mateer (1989) use 100% accuracy on three consecutive role plays, with no cueing on the last two days as a criterion of success.

Updating and Cleaning Routine

Each patient will be trained in the process of periodically removing old and unnecessary pages from their Memory Notebooks. So as to establish behavioral routines, it is recommended that the patient learn or be cued to complete this task on a designated day and will include updating the notebook to include next week's appointments as well as filing last week's log pages.

This sequence includes the following steps:
    a.   Remove old log sheets and place in file.
    b.   Put in the new log sheets for each day of the week and date them.
    c.   Double check your work.
    d.   Check the calendar (if appropriate) to see if there are any upcoming events. If so, they should be added to the Monday through Sunday pages on the weekly schedule page during the updating routine.

Scoring and Documentation

One possible system for recording performance is to have each therapist use the following scoring system:

4 — Patient independently recorded and retrieved all relevant activities and information during the session using the Memory Notebook.

3 — Patient needed minimum assistance to either record *or* retrieve information during the session using the Memory Notebook.

2 — Patient needed moderate assistance to record *and* retrieve information during the session using the Memory Notebook.

1 — Patient was unable to initiate utilization of the Memory Notebook.

The patient continues with this documentation until compliance is met, i.e., two consecutive weeks of complete/relevant documentation.

Training in the use of a Memory Notebook comprises the core of external memory strategies. However, it will often be necessary to supplement this training with the use of specific electronic devices, especially alarms, cell phones, or timers. These external compensations may be particularly important in cueing patients to use the notebook to complete a designated task at a designated time.

3.6 Memory Strategy Training

3.6.a. General Guidelines for Memory Strategy Training

Strategy training (sometimes referred to as "metacognitive strategy training" or "mnemonic strategy training" in the literature) refers to training the patient to use strategies or "mnemonics" that promote encoding and retrieval of information to be remembered without the use of external compensations. These strategies are typically internal and self-instructional strategies which can be either verbal or non-verbal, depending on the content of the information to be remembered, but can also be facilitated by external strategies, such as recording the mnemonic in a Memory Notebook.

Strategy utilization is based on explicit memory and self-instructional routines learned through cognitive rehabilitation. Strategy training is most effective for those with mild to moderate impairment of memory (Kaschel et al., 2002). Incorporating external compensations to assist with strategy utilization may be necessary if the patient's explicit memory is moderately impaired.

Other cognitive impairments may affect the extent to which the patient can utilize strategies in day-to-day life. Impairments of initiation, strategy generation, slow speed of information processing, or problems with visual imagery may determine the types of strategies used, and the extent to which they incorporate external compensations. Utilization of the previously discussed learning techniques such as errorless learning, spaced retrieval, or chaining may assist with the acquisition and retrieval of mnemonic strategies.

The clinician and patient together should determine in what situations the utilization of a mnemonic strategy is practically the most effective. The utilization of mnemonic strategies requires time for strategy generation and rehearsal based on anticipatory awareness of the need to use the strategy. In practical situations, sometimes it is simply easier to write the information down through a well-established procedural external compensation, especially of the information to be remembered needs only relatively short-term storage, e.g., a grocery list. On the other hand, utilization of mnemonic strategies for information that needs to be frequently available, such as the names of co-workers or relatives, may be most appropriate.

3.6.b Types of Memory Strategy Training

A variety of strategies appear in the evidence-based literature for the treatment of memory disorders. These strategies can be grouped into two major categories, including association techniques and organizational and elaboration techniques, as presented in Table 3-1. Within these major categories, specific strategies are noted in the following table, and are reviewed thereafter. Some of these strategies share characteristics of others, so each strategy is not necessarily exclusive of the other. Additionally, it is often appropriate and necessary to integrate the utilization of external compensations with strategy training.

Association Techniques

Association strategies are one of the most common strategies, where two or more items to be learned are linked or associated together. Visual-verbal and visual imagery have been used to learn and recall peoples' names. Accordingly, a name (verbal information) is linked with either a picture (visual) of the person or the image of a face (visual imagery). One technique using visual imagery was described by Wilson (2009) where the patient was taught to identify a prominent feature of the person's face which could be associated with their name. It is important for the patient to generate the potential association to promote the personal meaningfulness or relevance of the association. Other than visual associations, one might use a historical association based on previous experiences with that person, or affective association that capture the patient's feelings about that person.

Another example of using verbal-visual association for training memory of verbal information is through the utilization of visual schematics, which may convey the sequential or categorical relationship between information to be learned. For example, the following schematic provides for the opportunity to use a first letter mnemonic strategy, along with a visual schematic, to promote learning of a sequence of steps, which applies to the Goal-Plan-Do-Review (GPDR) approach to problem-solving as discussed in section 2.6.b.

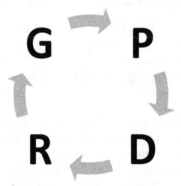

Visual imagery has been demonstrated to assist with the delayed recall of everyday relevant verbal material such as stories and appointments. In Kaschel et al. (2002, page 137-139), research outcomes revealed that use of imagery mnemonics were effective for mildly memory-impaired individuals. To initiate this strategy, patients are first introduced to examples of how they likely already use visual imagery to recall events.

Other variations of the association technique making use of visual imagery are the visual peg method (Wilson, 2009) and method of loci (West, 1995). These are primarily visual methods in which a list of several target items to be remembered is linked or associated with several key items/locations that are already known. These strategies require conscious planning and some level of creativity by the user, and are generally best used by individuals who have mild memory challenges.

In the visual peg method, the target items are linked with a standard set of peg words which are already learned and memorized in a fixed sequence. The literature describes use of a rhyming peg method; the classic example of this is one-bun, two-zoo (or shoe), three-tree, four-door, five-hive, and so on. Using this method, each target image to be learned is linked with one key image. The more interactive, silly or dynamic the visual associations are, the higher the likelihood the item will be successfully recalled. This strategy can be used functionally when someone may not be able to write down the information to be remembered. A functional example of use of this strategy would be remembering five grocery items to be purchased after viewing a posted flyer. The first item, bread, would be visually linked with "bun," hotdog buns would be visually linked with "zoo," and Gatorade would be visually linked with "tree," kiwis with "door", and finally Oreos with "hive." The patient is to visualize the two linked items interacting in some dynamic manner. After these associations are made, the patient can later retrieve the list by retrieving the previously learned rhymed word list with the associated visual image. This technique was utilized by a specific patient with the previous list by using these visual associations (many of these visual associations were also paired with a gesture by this patient):

1 — bun (bread) — slicing bread and placing beside buns.

2 — zoo (hotdog buns) — hotdog buns jumping up and down behind bars at a zoo.

3 — tree (Gatorade) — pouring Gatorade on the roots of a tree.

4 — door (kiwis) — smashing kiwis on the side of a door and seeing chunks of kiwi dripping off the door.

5 — hive (Oreos) — filling the spaces of a beehive with Oreo cookies.

Similarly, in the method of loci, target words are transformed into visual images and each image is mentally linked with a different location in a well-known place, e.g., one's bedroom or a frequented street. As the patient mentally scans through the room, the target items, which have been linked with a specific series of places or objects in the room, will be remembered. As with the visual peg method, the new items to be recalled are visually associated with the previously learned series of specific locations or objects in those locations.

Organizational Techniques

One of the most frequently used organizational techniques is to use the first letter of each of a series of words to form a single word or pseudo-word, simplifying the storage and retrieval of the information represented by that word. This organizational technique can be used for acquiring invariant knowledge that may be vocationally-relevant (e.g., "WEAP" — **W**ord, **E**xcel, **A**ccess and **P**owerPoint, each piece of software in Microsoft Office for a computer technician in training), or for information that is episodic in nature (e.g., your grocery list that day).

Patients can also be taught to use semantic clustering strategies to group information into clusters in order to enhance encoding and retrieval. Breaking the list into smaller informational categories, based on their semantics or meaning of the words, reduces the cognitive effort involved in the task. For example, a patient may use verbal clustering to remember shopping items in each section of a grocery store. To purchase eggs, lettuce, milk, pancake mix, butter, hamburger, blueberries, and onion, the patient may use the categories "fruits and vegetables," and "ingredients to make pancakes," as the two "clusters" of items. Another example of clustering could include clustering geographic destinations among a series of errands. If necessary, the utilization of mnemonic strategies can be combined with external compensation strategies, and the patient can write a grocery list based on these two categories.

Another organizational strategy that can be used for recall of more complex verbal and written information is the PQRST strategy (Glasgow, 1977; Wilson, 1987). The steps involved in the PQRST process are as follows:

1. **Preview:** Preview the information to be recalled.

2. **Question:** Ask key questions about the text (e.g., "What is the main point to be conveyed? In what year did the action take place? How many people were involved?")

3. **Read:** Read the material carefully to answer the questions.

4. **State:** State the answers and, if necessary, read the text again until it is possible to state the answers.

5. **Test:** Test regularly for retention of the information.

The PQRST strategy is essentially self-instructional, promotes active learning, and engages elaboration and review of what has been learned and remembered. Learning this strategy is, of course, particularly useful for patients returning to an academic environment.

Storytelling and humor are other mnemonic strategies that can assist recall of meaningful information. These strategies potentially add personal and emotional relevance to the information to be recalled, and may assist in associating information to be recalled with previous experiences that are well represented in memory. Creatively adding humor or jokes to the story promotes memory. Also, many patients find this activity pleasant and enjoyable, compared to their feelings about the frequent rehearsal and practice of cognitive tasks in which they are typically asked to engage.

3.6.c Stages of Strategy Training

Assessment and Selection of Techniques

There are a number of issues that must be taken into consideration when determining the most appropriate internal strategy and treatment plan. In particular, the following factors need to be assessed prior to initiating treatment:

1) The patient's cognitive strengths and weaknesses, to help determine whether a verbal or visual based approach is more appropriate.

2) The limits of the patient's capacity with respect to attention and working memory to determine how much information the patient can work with at any given time.

3) The extent of any accompanying impairments in awareness, motivation and/or executive functioning. If these difficulties are present, they will need to be addressed first or within the context of treatment.

Regardless of the technique being considered, it is essential to work collaboratively with the patient to identify his/her personal goals and future plans, and to help select training tasks that are meaningful to the patient. In order to maximize learning and promote eventual generalization, it is crucial to help identify what tasks are most important to the patient, as well as what learning strategies were previously used and already seem natural to them.

By the end of the assessment phase, the therapist should have identified the exact nature of the memory deficit, selected an appropriate technique to address the problem and determined whether verbal or visual methods will be used. Finally, appropriate, functional, and personally meaningful tasks will be selected to train the patient to use the strategy.

Acquisition Stage

During the acquisition stage, patients are introduced to the technique chosen to address their memory impairment. Therapists will typically begin with patient education regarding how learning the technique can improve their overall effectiveness and independence in performing their current everyday tasks. Examples and personal stories can help make the technique seem practical and useable. Patients can also be introduced to examples of how they have already used the technique in their own lives, to recall events, phone numbers, and/or other important information. This introduction provides motivation to build upon an already existing skill, rather than learning something completely novel.

Patients will also need to be taught the components and features of the chosen strategy and guided systematically through the steps involved in using it. By the end of this stage, the patient should be able to describe the methods involved in the technique, identify tasks and situations in which its use can help them, and be able to recite the steps involved in applying the strategy.

Application Stage

The application stage focuses on applying the technique to simple real-life and/or role-play tasks in context of their therapy. Examples may include learning therapists' names, the steps involved in various functional tasks such as transferring from a wheelchair to a bed, or their medication schedule.

Initially, high levels of external assistance and supervision are often needed, with the therapist providing specific instructions, modeling, coaching, and cues to assist the patient in applying the strategy. Ample practice and structure is given until the patient may become independent in applying the technique. Subsequently, the focus shifts to improving their accuracy in recalling the target information and with independent use of the strategy. This is achieved by gradually fading the level of therapist cueing and assistance.

Recall periods should start within sessions with increasing delays building from immediately after review, and increasing up to the end of the therapy session. Once the patient achieves 100% accuracy in recalling the target information during the treatment session, gradually increase the delay period across intervals of 24, 48, 72 hours, or even up to a week. Likewise, as the patient's accuracy increases, the therapist can also increase the amount and/or complexity of information to be remembered.

At the end of each session, the therapist records recall accuracy and the level of cueing required to use the strategy and to recall the target information. The therapist should also allow a few minutes during, or at the end of, each session to solicit the patient's opinion about their performance and to provide constructive feedback.

During the adaptation state, the clinician can and should model or cue strategy utilization for the patient. Patients must be able generate the technique themselves, thus making strategy utilization a self-generated process. The patient learns with practice to generate self-instructional questions, "How am I going to remember this?", to become independent with strategy generation and application. Once the patient achieves this goal, treatment can shift to focus on generalizing the technique to other tasks and settings.

Activities for Application Stage

1) Face/name association: Remembering names of the therapists or other patients.

2) Visual imagery: Recalling locations, such as how to get to the therapy room; remembering story details.

3) Verbal mnemonics: Remembering items on a mock grocery list, to-do lists; steps involved in functional activities (e.g., transferring).

4) Organizational strategy: Remembering one's medication schedule by category/purpose or administration time; organizing important details from a short newspaper or magazine article; remembering items from a mock grocery shopping list.

5) PQRST: Remembering information from a newspaper article or brief news programs.

Adaptation Stage

In this adaptation stage the patient begins to apply the techniques to more complex, functional, and everyday tasks outside the clinic or structured treatment environment. The focus is on promoting generalization of skills to problems that they will face in their everyday lives. The therapist's role here is largely supportive, with the goal of assisting them in determining which strategies are most appropriate and useful, and in identifying situations in which they can use the technique(s) in their daily lives outside the clinic. For example, if a patient is a student, the therapist might teach them how to use the PQRST method to improve overall study skills, as well as organizational strategies to help highlight and encode essential details to be remembered from texts.

There are a wide variety of tasks that can be utilized at this stage. Any task that was previously performed through in-clinic role playing can now be performed in the community. Examples include remembering details from lectures, articles, or vocational information, as well as prospective memory tasks, such as remembering pending appointments and events.

Because some internal memory strategies are more complex and/or time consuming than others, some are more amenable to generalization than others. Generalization does not occur automatically without cueing or monitoring from the therapist, and the patient will likely require assistance to maintain utilization of the strategy (Wilson, 1987). The following guidelines can help promote transfer of skills outside the therapy environment:

1) Focus on teaching strategies that the patient used naturally to help maximize the likelihood of generalization to other tasks and settings.

2) Help the patient identify how and when the use of the various techniques will be helpful for them.

3) When teaching patients to use mnemonics in their daily life, encourage them to generate their own. Information is more likely to be remembered when it is salient and personally meaningful.

4) Incorporate the family into treatment at this stage whenever possible, as they can play an important role in encouraging the patient to use the strategy in the home and community. Thus, even in situations where the patient does not spontaneously initiate using the technique, family members can remind them to apply and practice it in specific circumstances.

Activities for Adaptation Stage

1) Face/name association: Remembering names of classmates, co-workers, people at a party or other group gathering.

2) Visual imagery: Studying for a test: remembering pending appointments and events; remembering locations; recalling details about new people encountered.

3) Verbal mnemonics: To remember items from a grocery list when they go shopping in the community. Also to remember the steps involved in a recipe; lists when studying for tests; to-do lists.

4) Meeting people at a gathering: Clinician presents actual photographs of nonfamiliar faces/people, and provides five pieces of demographic information: first/last name, profession, and city/state. Patient then generates ideas of how to learn, but using the strategies presented. The level of difficulty can be increased by the number of informational elements to be recalled, and the rate in which the information is presented. To determine which strategies are the most successful for a patient, it can be very useful to ask the patient to indicate what strategy they are using when performing a given task and compare their performance according to different strategy utilization.

5) Organizational strategies: To help encode essential details from lectures and textbooks; remembering items from a grocery list by category (dairy, meat, frozen).

3.7 Complex Evidence-Based Programs for the Rehabilitation of Impairments of Memory

3.7.a Memory Rehabilitation Group

Thickpenny and Barker-Collo (2007) have provided evidence on the benefits of an eight-session group program, designed to teach memory strategies to patients with TBI and stroke. Each session is 60 minutes long and sessions are held twice weekly over four weeks. Material is presented using a combination of didactic teaching about memory and memory strategies, small group activities, discussions, problem-solving, and practice in implementing memory strategies.

The aims of the group are to: (1) explain what memory is and how it works; (2) assist participants in understanding their own memory impairment and its effects; (3) introduce and practice strategies to aid in memory and learning; and (4) assist participants to identify the most appropriate and useful strategies for them.

In each session, therapists review the previous session, present new information didactically, present daily life instructions, guide practices in strategy use and conduct group activities. Diaries, errorless learning, and rehearsal/repetition are also used throughout the course. Eight learning modules are described, as provided in Table 3-2:

Table 3-2 Memory Group Leaning Modules

Components of Memory Group Learning Modules (Thickpenny and Barker-Collo, 2007)	
Introduction: What is memory?	Definition of memory. Exercises to illustrate areas of memory. Defining three types of memory (e.g., sensory, short-term, long-term).
Model of memory	Defining the four components of memory: (attention, encoding, storage, retrieval). Introduction to flowchart linking types of memory to components of memory.
Attention and encoding	Defining attention and its subtypes. Illustrations from daily life and the impact of attention on memory functioning.
Strategies to improve attention	Identification and practice in the application of strategies geared to improve attention to information.
Encoding	Definition of encoding and its role in memory. Identification and practice of internal and external strategies to assist encoding.
Storage	Storage and its role in memory. Identification and practice of strategies to aid storage with emphasis on how to use a diary effectively.
Retrieval strategies	Identification of typical retrieval deficits. Identification, and practice of strategies to improve retrieval (e.g., word finding strategies).
Review	Final review of information from all the previous sessions.

(Reproduced from Thickpenny and Barker-Collo, 2007, by permission)

3.7.b TEACH-M

TEACH-M is a comprehensive instructional, theoretically motivated program, developed on empirical evidence from special education and neuropsychological rehabilitation research, to teach new skills to patients with moderate to severe cognitive impairments. It has been empirically supported by two recent studies (Sohlberg et al., 2005; Ehlhardt, 2005). Table 3-3 provides a summary of the components of TEACH-M.

Table 3-3 Components of TEACH-M

Task Analysis	Know the instructional content. Break up into small steps. Chain steps together.
Errorless Learning	Keep errors to a minimum during the acquisition phase. Model target steps before the patient attempts a new skill or step. Carefully fade support. If an error occurs, demonstrate the correct skill or step immediately and ask the client to do it again. Use simple, consistent instructional wording.
Assessment	Initial: assess skills before initiating treatment for the first time. Ongoing: probe performance at the beginning of each teaching session or before introducing a new step.
Cumulative review	Regularly integrate and review new skills with previously learned skills.
High rates of correct practice	Practice the skill several times. Distributed practice encourages this.
Metacognitive strategy	The prediction-reflection technique can be used to encourage active processing of the material or another appropriate strategy that encourages self-reflection and problem-solving.

(Reproduced from Ehlhardt et al., 2005, by permission)

3.8 Strategic and Tactical Goal Writing in Rehabilitation of Impairments of Memory

PATIENT LT: Goals for the use of an External Memory Notebook

Long-Term Strategic Goal:

Mr. LT will demonstrate daily use of his external memory device (e.g., planner) in his natural environments.

Monthly Strategic Treatment Goals

Possible Strategic Goal #1: Initiate/Continue _____ stage (e.g., acquisition, application, adaptation) of Memory Notebook strategy of memory protocol.

Possible Strategic Goal #2: Initiate/Continue _____ stage (e.g., acquisition, application, adaptation) of strategy for severe impairment of memory protocol.

Possible Strategic Goal #3: Initiate _____ stage (e.g., acquisition, application, adaptation) metacognitive strategy of the memory protocol.

Short-Term Tactical Treatment Goals:

STGa: Mr. LT will independently identify appropriate information for each section of his planner with 90% accuracy.

STGb: Mr. LT will independently find appropriate information efficiently in his planner by using the tab dividers with 90% accuracy.

STGc: Mr. LT will independently locate specific appointments on his daily schedule, including work, class and therapy times, through the addition of a permanent schedule area and use of the weekly planner section, with 90% independence.

STGd: Mr. LT will demonstrate emerging independent use of the planner outside of the therapy room by bringing the planner to 100% of the therapy sessions and increasing the number of entries made between therapy sessions.

PATIENT AZ: Goals for the use of an External Memory Notebook

Long-Term Strategic Goal

Mrs. AZ will set up a personal organizer and establish habits of its use to aid her in organizing and prioritizing appointments, personal information, and responsibilities for independent living.

Monthly Strategic Treatment Goals

Possible Strategic Goal #1: Initiate/Continue _____ stage (e.g., acquisition, application, adaptation) of Memory Notebook strategy of memory protocol.

Possible Strategic Goal #2: Initiate/Continue _____ stage (e.g., acquisition, application, adaptation) of strategy for severe impairment of memory protocol.

Possible Strategic Goal #3: Initiate _____ stage (e.g., acquisition, application, adaptation) metacognitive strategy of the memory protocol.

Short-Term Tactical Treatment Goals:

STGa: Mrs. AZ will purchase a personal organizer following clinician's specific recommendations.

STGb: Mrs. AZ will independently transfer appointments from all other calendars into the calendar section of her organizer within one week of purchase.

STGc: Mrs. AZ will independently transfer relevant names, addresses, and phone numbers into the contacts section of her organizer.

STGd: Mrs. AZ will record all pending appointments into her organizer at the time the appointment is made, with 100% accuracy.

STGe: Mrs. AZ will use her organizer while on the telephone, by recording specific information during 90% of opportunities.

STGf: Mrs. AZ will use the "To Do" section of the organizer to record tasks she needs to accomplish, and will refer to this list in order to structure her activities on a daily basis.

PATIENT DD: Goals for use of Complex Rehearsal Technique

Long-Term Strategic Goal

Mrs. DD will use strategies to improve her comprehension and retention of 2-4 paragraph length written text.

Short-Term Tactical Treatment Goals:

STGa: Mrs. DD will independently identify the steps of the PQRST (i.e., preview, question, read, summarize, test) reading method with 90% accuracy across two consecutive sessions.

STGb: Mrs. DD will complete the five PQRST steps with minimal clinician support when provided a 3-4 paragraph length text during the structured therapy session.

STGc: Mrs. DD will read 2-4 paragraph length texts of varying complexity (e.g., newspaper articles) and provide short answers to comprehension questions with 90% accuracy across two consecutive sessions.

STGd: Mrs. DD will independently complete and return homework provided between sessions demonstrating accurate use of the five PQRST steps with a 2-4 paragraph length text in 90% of opportunities.

PATIENT AF: Treatment Goals for the use of Spaced Retrieval

Long-Term Strategic Goal

Mrs. AF will produce accurate personal birth, date, and address when prompted.

Monthly Strategic Treatment Goals

Possible Strategic Goal #1: Initiate/Continue _____ stage (e.g., acquisition, application, adaptation) of Memory Notebook strategy of memory protocol.

Possible Strategic Goal #2: Initiate/Continue _____ stage (e.g., acquisition, application, adaptation) of strategy for severe impairment of memory protocol.

Possible Strategic Goal #3: Initiate _____ stage (e.g., acquisition, application, adaptation) metacognitive strategy of the memory protocol.

Short-Term Tactical Treatment Goals:

STGa: Given a clinician model of correct birth date or address, Mrs. AF will correctly repeat the information with 100% accuracy following a prompt question across two therapy sessions.

STGb: Mrs. AF will produce accurate personal birth, date, or address following delays of 15 seconds – 5 minutes, following a prompt question across two therapy sessions.

STGc: Mrs. AF will produce accurate personal birth, date, and address following delays of 5 -30 minutes following a prompt question across two therapy sessions.

STGd: Mrs. AF will produce accurate personal birth, date, and address following delays of up to 24 hours, following a prompt question across two therapy sessions.

STGe: Mrs. AF will independently produce accurate personal birth, date, and/or address in functional contexts (e.g. filling out medical form).

4. Rehabilitation for Impairments of Attention

4.1 Introduction

Deficits in attention are extremely common following acquired brain injury. Relatively subtle impairments in attention can significantly reduce a person's ability to function in day-to-day activities as attention is a foundational skill that underlies and supports all other cognitive abilities. As a result, attention deficits are an important target for efforts in cognitive rehabilitation.

Describing attention is complex as multiple scientific methods have been used to better understand it. Our understanding of attention comes from cognitive psychology, neurophysiology, and neuropsychology, among others. Essentially, how we describe attention is based on how we assess attention. Attention is comprised of a number of interrelated subprocesses. Over the years, several models of attention have been proposed. Some of these are based on an analysis of cognitive processing (Shiffrin & Schneider, 1977), others rely on neuroanatomic analyses of attention (Posner & Peterson, 1990), and still others on factor analytic research (Mirsky et al., 1991).

Sohlberg and Mateer (1987) have proposed a very useful clinical model of attention for the treatment of impairments of attention following brain injury and stroke. These authors divide attention into five hierarchically organized components: focused attention; sustained attention; selective attention; alternating attention; and divided attention.

Focused attention represents the most basic level of attention, and refers to the ability to recognize and acknowledge specific sensory information.

Sustained attention refers to the ability to maintain attention over a period of time during a continuous and repetitive activity. At the highest level, it includes mental control or working memory, by which one holds information in mind and performs some type of mental manipulation on it. Examples would be any simple cooking or typing task over a period of time in a relatively distraction free environment.

Selective attention is the ability to process target information selectively and inhibit responding to nontarget information, e.g., a student trying to focus on a teacher while ignoring the noise from the playground outside.

Alternating attention refers to the ability to shift one's focus between tasks or activities that demand different behavioral or cognitive skills. An example would be the work of a secretary who must switch between typing and answering phones.

Finally, divided attention refers to the ability to respond to two or more events or stimuli simultaneously. An example might be talking on the phone while doing the dishes, or driving on a busy highway, which requires monitoring one's speed and actively scanning the road.

4.2 Impairments of Attention after Brain Injury

Impairments of attention following brain injury are very diverse, and multiple types of impairments of attention frequently coexist in the same patient. The severity of impairment also varies significantly depending on the type, acuity, severity and location of injury. The heterogeneity of impairments in attention following brain injury therefore necessitate very individualized assessment and rehabilitation strategies and have challenged researchers in developing methodologies which control for this heterogeneity.

Almost any brain injury can result in impairment of attention. Impairments of focused attention and sustained attention are usually the result of subcortical injury including the brainstem and the ascending reticular activating system, the later of which includes especially the thalamus. The parietal lobes certainly contribute to the attentional system, and in the case of right parietal injury, the phenomena of neglect can be considered a sensory-specific example of an impairment of (spatial) attention. Impairment of higher levels of attentional processes, such as selective attention, alternating attention, and divided attention are often the result of frontal lobe impairment, or of structures on which the frontal lobes are depending for input (e.g., basal ganglia). Impairments of these higher level attentional processes often co-exist with impairment of executive functions. For these reasons, the rehabilitation of disorders of attention shares some common features with the rehabilitation of impairments of executive functions.

4.3 BI-ISIG Recommendations for the Rehabilitation of Impairments of Attention

In their most recent review of treatment interventions for attention, the BI-ISIG Cognitive Rehabilitation Task Force of ACRM has recommended, as a Practice Standard, remediation of attention during *post-acute* rehabilitation after TBI. Remediation of attention deficits after TBI should include direct attention training and strategy (metacognitive) training to promote development of compensatory strategies and foster generalization to real world tasks. However, there is still insufficient evidence to distinguish the effects of specific attention training during *acute* recovery and rehabilitation from spontaneous recovery, or from more general cognitive interventions (Cicerone et al., 2011).

Cicerone et al. (2011) cite three studies as examples of effective strategy training. In the first, Sohlberg et al. (2002) applied their Attention Process Training (APT) program to the rehabilitation of attention in patients with brain injury. In the second, Fasotti et al. (2000) used their Time Pressure Management program as a metacognitive strategy to learn skills to modulate the flow of information received, thereby avoiding attention overload. In the third, Cicerone (2002) provided strategy training in working memory skills in individuals with mild brain injury. Training included verbal mediation, rehearsal, anticipating task demands, self-pacing, and self-monitoring while performing working memory tasks. The results of these and similar studies also suggest that strategy training for attention provides greater benefits for complex tasks that require the regulation of attention, and fewer benefits for basic aspects of attention (e.g., reaction time or vigilance). This is consistent with the emphasis on strategy training, in the *post-acute* stage of recovery, to compensate for attention deficits in functional situations. The rehabilitation of attention includes some components of training reviewed in the chapters on rehabilitation of executive and memory disorders.

Based on emerging evidence, the BI-ISIG Cognitive Rehabilitation Task Force also recommended, as a Practice Option, that computer-based interventions may be considered as an adjunct to clinician-guided treatment for the remediation of attention deficits after traumatic brain injury or stroke (Cicerone et al., 2011). However, it was emphasized that the sole reliance on repeated exposure and practice on computer-based tasks without some involvement and intervention by a therapist was not recommended. The present work does not include computer-based strategies of attention training.

4.4 General Framework for the Rehabilitation of Impairments of Attention

Rehabilitation of impairments of attention that is based on the available evidence includes a variety of approaches to treatment, some that are unique to impairments of attention, but many also that integrate elements of strategies used in the treatment of impairments of executive and memory functions. The rehabilitation strategies include interventions that are designed to improve attentional processes (i.e., Attention Process Training) and others which incorporate strategy (metacognitive) training (i.e., Time Pressure Management and Working Memory).

The work of Sohlberg and colleagues represents the foundation for the rehabilitation of impairments of attention using Attention Process Training (APT). In their APT-II manual, Sohlberg and her colleagues list six basic principles in the treatment of cognitive impairment in general and attention deficits in particular (Sohlberg et al., 2001). These principles apply to each of the three approaches to attention training that are described in this manual.

1) Attention interventions should work from a theoretical model. A theory-driven approach ensures a meaningful rationale for the treatment approach being used. In the case of APT training, the model includes five components of attention: focused; sustained; selective; alternating; and divided. By providing a framework, the clinician can organize interventions and address the specific components that are impaired.

2) Task training needs to follow their hierarchical organization. It is important to provide repeated stimulation and activation of the foundational underlying process for facilitation of a new skill. As soon as a patient has mastered a foundational skill or has experienced recovery of function at a basic level, treatment moves on to higher level skills.

3) Repetition is essential. Repetition allows for a sufficient intensity of training which is considered critical for establishing an attention skill to the point that it becomes automatic.

4) Record-keeping of performance allows for data-based treatment. Careful records of performance during training allows the clinician to make informed decisions about when to start, stop, or modify a therapy program based on patient performance.

5) Attention training should include tasks to promote generalization of strategies. Many of the APT tasks tend to be laboratory-type tasks that allow for targeted, repetitive stimulation or practice of specific components of attention. Although research has tended to support this approach to attention training, the BI-ISIG recommendations emphasize the importance of supplementing these repetitive practice exercises with strategy training. Strategies to maximize attention abilities are learned and practiced during repetitive tasks, and practicing these strategies in other contexts is necessary for generalization.

6) The ultimate measures of success are improvements in real-world adaptation, including managing work and daily living or leisure time activities as opposed to improvements in therapy exercises or test scores.

Sohlberg and her colleagues also provide recommendations of a more general nature for "direct attention training" in the context of cognitive rehabilitation (Sohlberg et al., 2003). They suggest that direct attention training might be most helpful for *post-acute* or mildly injured patients with intact vigilance, as there is no evidence at this time to support the rehabilitation of impairments of vigilance. They also suggest using it in conjunction with strategy (metacognitive) training, including feedback, self-monitoring, and strategy training. In addition, they recommend using attention training at least once a week, as a part of an individualized program comprising a hierarchy of tasks that emphasize working memory, mental control, and selective, alternating, and/or divided attention.

4.5 Attention Process Training (APT) Training

The APT is a structured program of attention training consisting of five different tracks, corresponding to a hierarchically-organized, clinical theory of attention. This theory states that there are five major types of attention: focused, sustained, selective, alternating, and divided. This approach to the treatment of attention deficits has been empirically validated in a study by Sohlberg et al. (2000), in which the authors compared the efficacy of APT with that of brain-injury education. They found APT to enhance performance on a number of functional tasks and neuropsychological measures of executive attention and working memory. Subjects also showed gains in self reported attention ability.

APT-I is for patients with significant impairment, and APT-II for those whose impairments are less severe. The following information is drawn exclusively from these sources. Therapists who intend to work with the APT program will need to read and learn the material contained in the APT manuals.

The initial stage of APT training focuses on a thorough assessment of the problem. Assessment can involve either formal neuropsychological testing, self-report measures, or behavioral rating scales. The goal is to identify the specific type of attention impairment (i.e., focused, sustained, selective, alternating, divided), as well as the tasks at home, work, or in the community that will be targeted for generalization.

The APT-II includes a brief test of attention, the "Attention Process Training Test." It also includes a structured questionnaire and attention rating scales. The APT-II Attention Questionnaire explores the presence of deficits in the different areas of attention, and can be used to inform the creation of an individualized training plan. Another measure, the Attention Log, can be used by patients or clinicians to record breakdowns or successes in attention activities, both initially in the assessment phase and throughout the course of therapy.

The "APT Test" will identify which of the five areas of attention are functioning suboptimally. Treatment should initially focus on the most fundamental or basic area of attention in which a person has difficulty. Each of the five tracks in the APT training corresponds to one of the five types of attention impairment. Within each of these tracks are a number of separate exercises and tasks arranged hierarchically in order of difficulty. Patients will work in the tracks that reflect their particular deficits and generally begin with those tasks that are most elementary. As they experience success, they proceed to tasks that are more complex.

In their manuals, the authors note that treatment is highly individualized and is difficult to apply in a group setting. In addition, within each of the five tracks, there may be some trial and error in choosing tasks and schedules, and the patient's performance will provide the data necessary to tailor an individualized program.

The APT program makes use of a variety of quantitative and qualitative measures along with the appropriate scoring and documentation forms. Quantitative measures record the accuracy, speed, or level of cueing needed for task completion. Qualitative measures assess various clinical impressions including specific patterns of errors, patient factors that could impact or reflect performance (e.g., fatigue, depression, anxiety, pain, distractibility, etc.), and/or environmental factors (e.g., noise, temperature, interruptions, etc.). As patients improve, either quantitatively or qualitatively, they can progress to more difficult tasks within the targeted tracks.

APT focuses on generalization throughout training, with particular emphasis on transferring strategies to novel contexts in the final stage of treatment. In the manual, the authors provide very useful information on generalization strategies in attention and, in fact, recommend planning for generalization tasks even before therapy begins (Sohlberg et al., 2001).

The authors offer guidelines for designing generalization activities for each of the identified areas of impairment. To set up a generalization program, they recommend initially observing function in naturalistic settings to assess baseline performance. These observations enable the clinician to select generalization tasks which address the area of impaired attention. In therapy sessions, the patients work on discrete APT tasks in each of their targeted areas. Subsequently, but before the patient begins to implement generalization activities, more naturalistic probes are taken. Finally, patients are trained in the rationale, schedule, and logistics of performing the generalization tasks and filling out the related forms and data sheets.

4.5.a APT Generalizing Activities
(from Sohlberg, M.; Johnson, L.; Paule, L.; Raskin, S.; and Mateer, C. 2001)

Sustained Attention

Residential

1) Cooking
2) Paying bills/balancing checkbook
3) Child care
4) Cleaning/housekeeping
5) Car maintenance
6) Writing letters/correspondence
7) Constructional hobbies/handicrafts

Vocational

1) Typing
2) Answering phone calls
3) Adding figures; doing inventory
4) Stocking shelves
5) Documentation/paperwork
6) Building/construction activities
7) Data entry tasks

Community Settings

1) Driving
2) Grocery shopping
3) Banking
4) Library
5) Completing list of errands
6) Recreational activities
7) Fitness activities

Alternating Attention

Residential

1) Cooking while monitoring the washer/dryer cycles
2) Balancing checkbook with periodic phone interruptions
3) Housecleaning chore with child care responsibilities (e.g., periodic monitoring of children's play)
4) Car maintenance with frequent interruptions

Vocational

1) Switching between phone and typing task
2) Construction task requiring switching between reading plans or instructions and assembly
3) Adding figures; doing inventory/data entry with frequent interruptions
4) Stocking shelves with frequent interruptions

Community Settings

1) Transportation task requiring walking and consulting map
2) Banking errand with multiple components (e.g., deposit, withdrawal, getting balance)
3) Exercise program at gym requiring use of multiple machines.
4) Completing list of errands

Selective Attention

Residential

1) Cooking tasks with children playing in the background
2) Household chores with TV or radio playing
3) Doing jigsaw puzzles while other conversation is ongoing in room
4) Woodworking task with ongoing machine noise

Vocational

1) Filling out paperwork in busy office
2) Taking inventory of shelves in noisy, busy warehouse
3) Assembly line production with music playing in workroom
4) Work duties in office with lots of traffic going by window

Community Settings

1) Eating at busy, loud cafeteria
2) Doing series of small errands at busy mall
3) Following score and plays at baseball or football game
4) Going to a fair, picnic, festival, etc. and participating in food or game activity

Divided Attention

Residential

1) Cooking task with two items requiring simultaneous monitoring
2) Talking on the phone while doing the dishes

Vocational

1) Taking written minutes during a work meeting (i.e., simultaneous listening and writing tasks
2) Operating machinery which requires monitoring multiple dials or systems at the same time

Community Settings

1) Driving on a freeway or busy highway
2) Playing video games at arcade which require divided attention

(Reproduced from Sohlberg et al., 2001, by permission)

4.6 Time Pressure Management

Time Pressure Management (TPM) is a training strategy designed to assist patients to deal more effectively with the mental slowness that can produce cognitive overload and impair functioning. Individuals with brain injury frequently demonstrate slowed information processing, and have particular difficulty processing information under pressure or time constraints. Patients are instructed to apply a structured problem-solving strategy to assist them in the control and regulation of information input (Fasotti et al., 2000). As such, TPM incorporates elements of techniques used in the rehabilitation of executive and memory disorders.

A useful guide to training patients in the use of Time Pressure Management has recently been published (Winkens, Van Heugten, Fasotti, & Wade, 2009). TPM trains patients to make effective decisions both before and during the execution of a task. For example, before beginning a task it is often helpful to develop a long-term plan to compensate for and minimize problems, in this case mental slowness. These are referred to as "strategic" decisions. Then, during the execution of a task, patients often must make somewhat more short-term, moment-to-moment adjustments to avoid problems. These adjustments, referred to as "tactical" decisions, can reduce or prevent subsequent problems when carrying out the task.

However, such planning and short-term adjustments may not work, requiring many more rapid decisions, under time pressure, when encountering problems during the task. These are referred to as actions at the "operational" level. In the management of cognitive slowness, such actions reflect attempts to manage attention demands in the moment, under what may be severe time pressure conditions. TPM as a treatment strategy incorporates components of all three levels of decision making: the strategic; the tactical; and the operational. In addition, the authors describe training as taking place in three distinct stages: identifying the problem; teaching the strategy; and generalization.

4.6.a Stage 1: Identifying the Problem

In stage one of TPM training, the therapist assesses patients' subjective impressions of the problem and their objective performance on a number of tasks. To do this, neuropsychological testing might be helpful in addition to more specific measures of cognitive speed. Two such measures have been developed by Winkens, Van Heugten, Fasotti, and Wade (2009). The Mental Slowness Observation Test, a subjective measure, is a self-report rating scale comprising 21 items that reflect speed of information processing. The Mental Slowness Questionnaire is an objective semi-structured observational measure of four tasks: (1) following instructions on a route; (2) obtaining train times by telephone; (3) sorting money; and (4) looking up telephone numbers. The explicit goals of pre-treatment assessment are: (1) to establish an accurate picture of patient's attention skills and cognitive speed; and (2) increase patients' awareness of their problems.

4.6.b Stage 2: Teaching the Strategy

In stage two of the training process, patients are taught to use the TPM strategy, and implement it in a process that reflects the four primary steps of problem-solving: awareness of the problem; anticipation and planning; execution and self-monitoring; and self-evaluation.

First, the patient is trained to recognize, through education and feedback, that mental slowness is present and is having a demonstrable effect on performance. This can lead to certain situations of information overload, in which there are typically two or more things to be done at the same time for which there is not enough time (e.g., write information down while listening to it). Second, the patient is taught to develop a short plan to avoid such situations using strategic and tactical planning. Third, the patient makes an emergency plan describing what to do in case of overwhelming time pressure. Fourth, the patient attempts to carry out the plan and monitors its success in dealing with the time pressure problem. Table 4-1 provides the stages and components of TPM training (Van Heugten, Wade, & Fasotti, 2009).

Table 4-1   Stages, Components and Prerequisites for TPM

STAGES	COMPONENTS	PREREQUISITES	TREATMENT
STAGE 1: **Identifying the Problem**	Diagnosis of mental slowness Patient accepting the problem	Awareness of therapist Awareness of patient	Neuropsychological Testing Mental Slowness Questionnaire Mental Slowness Observation Test Feedback and demonstration Practice, explanation and feedback
STAGE 2: **Teaching the Strategy**	Patient learning the strategy Analyze the task for time pressure Make a plan of decisions and actions to undertake before the task starts Make an emergency plan Execute the task and monitor Apply the strategy	Anticipatory awareness and emergent awareness Sufficient learning ability Adequate cognitive skills Enough rest Sufficient motivation Patient should agree that it works Awareness that the strategy is a general one that can be be applied to other situations.	Distributed practice Meaningful and personalized Information and examples Practice, feedback and demonstration
STAGE 3: **Generalization**	Apply the strategy in new and more difficult situations	Sufficient cognitive skills	Practice, feedback and demonstration

(Reproduced from Winkens et al., 2009, by permission)

Patients are trained to memorize the four steps in the TPM problem-solving process before practice begins, and are frequently reminded of them throughout training. Specific strategies taught in the context of Time Pressure Management are: (1) asking for more specific information; (2) asking for more specific instructions; (3) asking if the other person can briefly stop talking, for example when verbal instructions are being given; (4) making a written plan on how to perform a task; and (5) restating the most important instructions. More generally, the patient is taught skills in verbal mediation, rehearsal, anticipation of task demands, self-pacing, and self-monitoring. As mentioned, these strategies have been addressed in Chapter 2 on executive functions, but are addressed in the present chapter as the strategies are provided for the treatment of disorders of attention. Table 4-2 provides examples of TPM (Winkens et al., 2009).

Table 4-2 Plans and Emergency Plans for TPM

EXAMPLE 1: Driving a car	Before leaving: study the route so that no decisions have to be made or discussions have to be held while driving; leave on time, so that you will not have to hurry, or worry that you will be late. During driving: turn off the radio so that you will not be distracted; ask passengers not to distract you with difficult conversations and ask them to help you watch road signs etc.; keep ample distance from the cars in front of you so that you can see what is happening further along the road, so you have enough time to react; do not drive too fast.	In case of panic or overwhelming time pressure: move the car to the side of the road and stop. Take a break, then take another look at your plan and your preventing decisions and actions, and use them!
EXAMPLE 2: Cooking a meal	Before starting to cook: read the recipe thoroughly, so that you know what has to be done in which order, and how much time it will take you to cook the meal; decide which things can be done first before turning on the stove; open cans and wrappings and put everything within arm's reach; wash the vegetables and cut them; turn off the phone to prevent distraction. During cooking: do not be distracted by other things; do not leave the stove to watch television or read a magazine when you have to wait a few minutes (for example, when waiting for pans to reach boiling point).	In case of panic or overwhelming time pressure: when the door bell rings, turn off the cooker, and then answer the door. When you have to take care of two things at the same time (for example you have to pour the water off the pasta, and turn the meat over to prevent it from burning), turn off the cooker, take the pasta off the stove, pour the water off, and then start again with the meat.
EXAMPLE 3: Retrieving information at a travel agency	Before going to the agency: make a list of all the things you would like to know. At the agency: read through your questions while waiting for your turn; ask the employee to take you to a quiet room so that you will not be distracted, and will not feel the urge to hurry because of the queue of people behind you. During the conversation: make notes; ask the employee to speak slowly so that you can keep up with him or her	In case of overwhelming time pressure: ask for repetition or more information when things are not clear. Ask the employee to write the important things down for you. Ask for a pause to review your questions. Did you get a satisfying answer to every question?

(Reproduced from Winkens et al., 2009, by permission)

As the newly-learned strategy is applied to specific tasks and situations, Winkens et al. (2009) offer a number of recommendations. These include: (1) initially targeting those tasks that are relatively easy; (2) starting treatment by first modeling the strategy for the patients, and then having them use an overt self-talk method to talk themselves through the task; (3) frequently reminding patients of the need to learn the importance of using the strategy to avoid failure; and (4) using a distributed practice paradigm in which brief learning trials are spread out over a long period of time (rather than crowded together into a longer learning trial).

In addition, different types of role-plays or tapes can be used in the training. For example, a therapist can give directions to a location and the patient is asked to repeat what the person said. In another, a therapist gives instructions on how to do a computer task. In each case, the patient is to apply the TPM strategy to maximize utilization and recall of the information.

One goal of treatment is to enable a patient to use the strategy independently, without prompts or overt guidance from the therapist. For example, patients can be trained to look for internal or external warning signs of time pressure to enhance emergent awareness. Internal signs could be feelings of panic, confusion, or tension. External signs could be the comments or actions of others that suggest the patient is having difficulty understanding or following the conversation. Such training may help patients recognize when to use the strategy. These signs become a cue for the patient to implement a TPM strategy.

For a variety of reasons, some patients will not be able to implement TPM strategies independently. For example, some individuals may not accurately read situations and thereby know when to implement the strategy. Others may be able to see the need, but be unable to remember planned solutions (at the strategic or tactical levels), or successfully implement them. For these individuals, training may need to emphasize the need to always use the strategy in certain situations or on certain tasks, with the assumption that it will usually be necessary and helpful.

4.6.c Stage 3: Generalization

In stage three, patients are trained to generalize the TPM strategy to other settings and tasks. To do this, they can be trained on a variety of tasks and in a number of different settings that are relevant to his or her life and interests, similar to what was described for APT (see section 4.5.a *APT Generalizing Activities*).

4.7 Rehabilitation of Working Memory

Cicerone (2002) investigated the effectiveness of improving attention by addressing underlying problems with working memory. Attention problems were viewed as reflecting problems with the temporary maintenance and manipulation of mental representations. These tend to be more pronounced in situations which demand attention to rapidly presented information and/or multiple sources of information.

In this study, subjects were taught to use strategies to allocate attention resources and manage the rate of information processing. Similar to studies with APT, these subjects were given hierarchically organized working memory tasks to improve complex attention skills. However, unlike APT, the focus was on strategic (metacognitive) training for impairments of attention. The intervention was based on the *n-back* procedure.

The *n-back* task has previously been used to examine the neural basis of the central executive component of working memory. The general *n-back* procedure consists of the presentation of a sequence of stimuli with the requirements for the participant to continuously report the stimulus occurring *n* number of stimuli previously. For example, in the *1-back* condition, a set of digits are presented sequentially in random order and the participant is instructed to report the digit which occurred one prior to the current digit. The *2-back* condition also consists of a randomly ordered sequence of digits, however the participant is now instructed to report the digit which occurred once removed from (or two prior to) the digit currently presented. While this paradigm can be presented using various modalities and protocols, the current treatment procedure was implemented with the use of common playing cards as a means of presenting the stimuli. This was done for two reasons. First, it was felt that the use of playing cards would provide a familiar, nonthreatening context for the treatment participants. Secondly, the manual presentation of stimuli allowed the therapist to quickly and easily modify conditions of the task, such as changing from self-paced to externally-paced presentation or reviewing previously viewed stimuli. Three variants of the basic *n-back* task were presented.

4.7.a LEVEL I. *N-Back* Procedures

I. 1-Back: Place sample cards one at a time a in horizontal line while explaining to the patient to name the card once removed from the card being placed, e.g.,:

> *Stimulus:*   2 5 7 9 8 ...
>
> *Response:*   – 2 5 7 ...

Then continue placing cards, this time in a single pile so that each previous card is covered and only the top card is showing. Allow the patient to ask questions and practice in this manner until they can perform two consecutive correct responses.

I. Instruct the patient to, *"Now do the same thing for this whole set, naming the card that is one back, working at your own pace, but try to go through this deck as accurately and efficiently as you can. Give me an answer for every card, even if you are not sure. If you miss one, just try to get back on track and do the best you can.* Have the patient place cards in order while naming the card *once removed*. Record responses and total time."

II. 2-Back. Repeat instructions as in part I, this time illustrating the procedure for naming the card *twice removed* (2-back) e.g.,:

> *Stimulus:*   2 5 7 9 8 ...
>
> *Response:*   – – 2 5 7 ...

II. Instruct patient to *Now do the same thing for this whole set, naming the card that is two back, working at your own pace, but try to go through this deck as accurately and efficiently as you can. Give me an answer for every card, even if you are not sure. If you miss one, just try to get back on track and do the best you can.* Have the patient place cards in order while naming the card *twice removed*. Record responses and total time.

In clinical practice, the administration can be varied by having the therapist place the cards and changing the rate of stimulus presentation, as well as allowing the patient to place the cards at his or her own pace. These variations allow the therapist to make observations and inferences regarding the impact of rate of information processing demands on performance. The patient can also be allowed to stop, review and correct errors as part of the intervention, in order to illustrate and emphasize how the patient may control aspects of performance and regulate their attention, particularly with regards to error monitoring.

Additional manipulations can be introduced (using either 1-back or 2-back methods, or moving between them). For example:

A) Patient is asked to name both the number and color of the *n-back* stimulus. This introduces a 'complex' stimulus situation requiring encoding of more than one stimulus attribute. This usually represents only a slight increase in difficulty for most patients. The patient can also be instructed to shift between the color and number stimulus attribute on alternating cards, or randomly according to the therapist's prompt.

B) The patient is asked to name the color of the card that is face up, **prior** to naming the number of the *n-back* card. This introduces the concept of "interruptions" to performance (internal or external) and the task of maintaining information in working memory while responding to an intervening demand.

C) The patient is asked to generate a response at random points during the *n-back* procedure (e.g., providing examples of items from a category (e.g., "name a fruit") or processing elements of a stimulus (e.g., "How many letters in the word 'orange' ? "). This continues to address the ability to "place mark" and maintain information in working memory while responding to distractions or interruptions, emphasizing the subject's ability to regulate their attention.

III. Working memory — Sorting Task. Another set of thirty-eight playing cards from all four suits are presented, and participants were required to sort the cards into four piles by suit while simultaneously reporting the *n-back* card value. The patient should be instructed to sort the cards by suit, placing each card in a pile beneath the cue card that is provided, while simultaneously naming the card *once* or *twice* removed from the last card placed down in any pile. Thus, there are four card values showing at any time, and the card value which was to be named can either be exposed or covered by another card at different sequences in the sort. Observation of variant of the task suggests that the additional exposed cards may serve as a source of potential interference, which has to be monitored and controlled by the patient. This version of the task can again be experimenter- or self-paced.

4.7.b LEVEL II. *N-Back* with Additional Working Memory Demands (random generation)

The primary *n-back* tasks are identical to those described above. In addition, participants are required to make a self-generated response on each trial, prior to naming the relevant card in the *n-back* task. This condition is introduced to further increase demands upon working memory and, specifically, to simulate the functional requirement of internally generating a response while maintaining a mental representation which would facilitate resumption of the (external) *n-back* task. Two variants of this condition have been employed, based upon a random generation procedure. Random generation is a technique that is also believed to tap the functions of the central executive, and has previously been employed to assess working memory in persons with TBI. In the first condition, participants are required to generate an example from two or more semantic categories, without repeating examples from the same category on successive trials. In the second condition, participants are required to generate a random letter triad (e.g., AKU) without using examples which represent words, natural letter sequences, or acronyms. The subject is asked to respond, prior to the naming the *n-back* stimulus, with three "random letters. Random letters require that the letters are not in alphabetic order (e.g., ABC), are not acronyms (e.g., USA or HBO) and are not words (e.g., CAT).

4.7.c LEVEL III. *N-Back* with Continuous Secondary Task

At this level of intervention the patient engages in an ongoing secondary task while maintaining performance on the primary *n-back* task and actively allocating attentional resources between the various task demands. This condition was introduced to simulate the occurrence of interrupting an ongoing activity in order to respond to an additional task, while maintaining a mental representation of the primary task, which would allow one to return to the original activity. The secondary tasks can be individually tailored in an effort to replicate a relevant aspect of each participant's real-life demands. For example, in the case of one patient who was required to participate in conference phone calls and negotiate the needs of several clients as part of her work responsibilities, the secondary task consisted of shadowing audiotaped lectures and conversations. Another patient whose work required him to look up serial numbers from an inventory and enter these numbers into another database for requisitions, was required to perform an ongoing, written clerical task to determine if two numbers and names were identical.

4.7.d Clinical Application

The intervention is typically provided as an individual treatment in one-hour sessions. Within each one-hour session, at least 20 to 30 minutes are typically devoted to feedback and discussion of the participant's performance, identification of task variables which influenced performance, development of strategies for effective task performance, management of secondary emotional responses during task performance (e.g., frustration) especially insofar as these reactions interfered with cognitive performance, identification and analysis of relevant attentional difficulties in the person's everyday functioning, and facilitating the application of within-session strategies to everyday functioning. While treatment should be individually tailored to reflect participants' clinical needs, there were several common themes. For example, initial treatment sessions are typically directed toward providing the participants with an interpretation of their attention deficits and a rationale for the intervention. The impact of slowed processing speed on performance is discussed, particularly the interrelationship between attention capacity and processing speed. The relationship between attention difficulties and subjective symptoms such as irritability and fatigue may also be explored in cognitive rehabilitation, where observations during training may serve as a basis for the therapist to explore, interpret or "explain" the impact of attention difficulties on other, noncognitive symptoms. For example, limitations in capacity to hold information or process multiple pieces of information may relate to an instance where the person becomes irritable (e.g., too much stimulation). The patient's experience of a need to marshal extra effort to meet attention demands may contribute to mental fatigue. Careful observation and constructive feedback during cognitive rehabilitation can, and should, provide the opportunity to promote the patient's awareness and behavioral self-regulation.

Subsequent treatment sessions are directed at facilitating the participants' conscious and deliberate use of strategies to effectively allocate attentional resources and manage the rate of information. Verbal mediation, rehearsal, anticipation of task demands, and self-pacing strategies should be introduced and practiced by the treatment participants throughout the various training tasks. Self-paced trials should be timed, and feedback can be provided regarding the relationship between pace and errors during task performance, as well as the need to utilize different strategies during self-paced and therapist-paced trials. During self-paced dual task trials, the participants can be allowed to pause one activity to reinforce the self-management of time demands. Participants are often asked to self-monitor their level of "effort" during performance, and this can be related to task variations and objective indices of performance. Participants are encouraged and reinforced for maintaining task performance even when frustrated, and the use of positive self-statements for management of emotional reactions is recommended. Aversive emotional reactions and "intrusive worrying" by participants over their performance can be interpreted as an additional cognitive demand which utilizes limited resources, tapping into the same underlying brain mechanisms, and thereby exacerbating or contributing to attentional difficulties. It is common to incorporate clinical interventions to help participants manage their emotional reactions or feelings of being overwhelmed by the demands on their attention.

During response generation and dual-task trials, participants are initially instructed to maintain their performance on the primary task while 'sharing' resources; on some occasions, however, participants can be instructed to place priority on the 'secondary' task, or to shift priorities between primary and secondary tasks within a trial. Participants frequently monitor the occurrence of 'attention lapses' during daily activities between treatment sessions, including the precipitating situation and use of strategies to regulate attentional resources and manage attentional demands. The later treatment sessions, especially during the dual-task trials, are increasingly devoted to fostering the participants' self-appraisal and application of strategy use in the context of their everyday functioning. Overall, an integral aim of the treatment is to increase participants' control over the allocation of attention resources and manage potential secondary consequences of reduced attention (e.g., fatigue, irritability, feeling overwhelmed) in their daily functioning.

4.8 Strategic and Tactical Goal Writing in Rehabilitation of Impairments of Attention

PATIENT XX: Goals for Time Pressure Management Training

Long-Term Strategic Goal

Mr. XX will consistently implement time pressure management strategies in the home environment for complex, multi-step task completion.

Monthly Strategic Treatment Goal

Initiate/Continue _____ stage (e.g., acquisition, application, adaptation) of time pressure management training strategy.

Short-Term Tactical Treatment Goals

STGa: Following clinician review and moderate verbal cueing, Mr. XX will state the four steps for managing complex situations.

STGb: Given functional scenarios of complex situations in written or auditory presentation, Mr. XX will write the steps with minimum clinician support.

STGc: Given functional scenarios of complex situations in written or auditory presentation, Mr. XX will state the steps for task completion with use of a visual aid.

STGd: Given functional scenarios of complex situations in written or auditory presentation, Mr. XX will independently state the steps for task completion.

STGe: In functional role-play scenarios in a clinical setting, Mr. XX will demonstrate appropriate application of the steps in 80% of opportunities.

STGf: Mr. XX will report on a provided tracking sheet, three instances weekly when the time pressure management steps were applied when completing functional activities at home.

PATIENT JK: Goals and Strategies for Attention Training

Long Term Strategic Goal

Mr. JK will improve his sustained, selective, and divided attention skills to increase his safety and to facilitate optimal performance on cognitive and functional tasks.

Monthly Strategic Treatment Goal:

Initiate/Continue _____ stage (e.g., acquisition, application, adaptation) of goals and strategies for attention training.

Short-Term Tactical Treatment Goals

STGa: Mr. JK will perform large shape cancellation tasks with 75% accuracy.

STGb: Mr. JK will perform double simultaneous large-shape cancellation tasks with 100% accuracy.

STGc: Mr. JK will perform double simultaneous small-shape cancellation tasks with 75% accuracy.

STGd: Mr. JK will perform small number cancellation tasks with distracter overlay and 90% accuracy.

STGe: Mr. JK will locate 3/5 small objects in a cluttered drawer with minimal clinician assistance.

STGf: Mr. JK will independently locate 5/5 targets on semi-complex maps.

STGg: Mr. JK will perform flexible shape cancellation tasks with 90% accuracy.

PATIENT EE: Goal and Strategies for Attention Training

Long Term Strategic Goal

Mrs. EE will demonstrate 90% accuracy on functional reading and writing tasks in a structured clinical setting with auditory distraction, to improve attention during completion of home activities.

Monthly Strategic Treatment Goal

Initiate/Continue _____ stage (e.g., acquisition, application, adaptation) of goals and strategies for attention training.

Short-Term Tactical Treatment Goals

STGa: Mrs. EE will respond with 90% accuracy to multiple choice comprehension questions to 1-2 paragraph narratives with TV news background.

STGb: Mrs. EE will respond with 90% accuracy to written two-step math story problems with TV news background.

STGc: Mrs. EE will assemble a 4-6 step recipe with 90% accuracy with natural environmental noise distraction.

STGd: Mrs. EE will independently complete a sample bill paying activity with 90% accuracy with natural environment noise distraction.

5. Rehabilitation of Hemispatial Neglect

5.1 Introduction

Hemispatial neglect represents a significant challenge for the patient and rehabilitation professionals. Patients with neglect are typically unaware of this impairment, especially in the acute phase of recovery. The rehabilitation of hemispatial neglect must therefore sometimes incorporate elements from the chapter on the rehabilitation of executive functions (see section 2.7.b). Research on the rehabilitation of hemispatial neglect has demonstrated that systematic training in visual scanning, sometimes accompanied by either real or imagined motor activity of the left arm or hand, is effective in improving neglect.

5.2 Hemispatial Neglect in Brain Dysfunction

Patients with lesions in the right cerebral hemisphere often show a reduced tendency to respond to and actively search for objects in the contralateral side of space, even though they may have intact visual fields on ophthamological testing. This is most commonly referred to as hemispatial neglect, unilateral neglect, or hemi-inattention. A significant number of patients with right hemisphere injury present with neglect in the acute stage, and while many improve, chronic visual neglect can have a dramatic effect on daily activities, even those that are basic such as eating, grooming, dressing, or reading. Hemispatial neglect for visual information is sometimes accompanied by impairments of attention to tactile and proprioceptive, as well as auditory, stimuli on the contralateral side of the injury.

5.3 BI-ISIG Recommendations for Hemispatial Neglect

The BI-ISIG Cognitive Rehabilitation Task Force of ACRM has recommended, as a Practice Standard (Cicerone et al., 2011), visuospatial rehabilitation that includes visual scanning training for left visual neglect after right hemisphere stroke. Limb activation or electronic technologies for visual scanning training may be included in the treatment of neglect after right hemisphere stroke as a Practice Option. Also, systematic training of visuospatial deficits and visual organization skills, without visual neglect, may be considered a Practice Option for persons with visual perceptual deficits after right hemisphere stroke as part of acute rehabilitation.

5.4 General Framework for the Rehabilitation of Hemispatial Neglect

Since the 1960's, researchers have made efforts to establish effective treatment for left neglect. Initial studies in this area focused primarily on the use of visual scanning strategies, including "anchoring" and training patients to look to the left. In the earliest published work in this area, researchers at NYU Langone Medical Center, Rusk Institute of Rehabilitation Medicine, conducted a series of studies to improve scanning capability in individuals with right brain damage (RBD), hoping to ameliorate the left neglect and visual inattention caused by the stroke. In an initial study (Weinberg et al., 1977), 57 patients with visual perceptual problems following RBD were randomly assigned to either a treatment group ($n = 25$) receiving 20 hours of scanning training across four weeks, or a control group ($n = 32$) that did not receive the training. Both groups participated in conventional occupational therapy over the four-week period. Following training, the experimental group improved on four visual academic tasks e.g., reading and arithmetic, while the control group did not. More severely-impaired patients showed greater improvement when compared with their controls, than did the more mildly-impaired group when compared with their controls.

In another representative study, Pizzamiglio et al. (1992) provided visual scanning training to a group of 13 RBD patients with left visual neglect. Patients ranged from 3-34 months post-stroke, and received training five times a week for eight weeks. Following training, all but one patient demonstrated improvement on a variety of impairment-based and functional tasks and this improvement appeared to be independent of spontaneous recovery. Most importantly, treatment gains generalized to functional tasks at home and were especially evident on tasks requiring exploratory scanning and sequential analysis of multiple target stimuli. However, training did not generalize to all visuo-spatial tasks and improvement did not occur in the one patient whose unawareness of his impairment did not resolve. Moreover, all patients continued to show variability in their neglect as a function of the density of the visual display and salience of the objects in their right visual field.

Diller and associates at Rusk hypothesized that the visual perceptual deficits in RBD suggested a typology: (a) patients with RBD may display gross disturbance in left to right scanning and neglect of most stimuli in the left side of space; (b) patients may present with additional disturbances of sensory awareness and spatial organization; or (c) patients may demonstrate a lateral visual field inattention only under more cognitively challenging task demands (Gordon et al., 1984; Weinberg et al., 1977). In a follow-up study to the one mentioned above (Weinberg et al., 1979), the research group added training in sensory awareness and spatial organization to the scanning protocol, and trained 30 patients with RBD using a two-phase treatment program. Fifteen hours were spent on scanning training using a visual tracking device to follow a moving target and search for lights on a board, as well as practice in visual cancellation tasks and reading. Five hours were then spent in training: (a) sensory awareness, using a mannequin, whereby the patient was touched on the back (using grid-marked locations) and was asked to identify the same locations on the back of a mannequin; and (b) spatial organization by using plexiglass cylinders of different lengths to estimate size differences on and off the body. The experimental group improved more than the (20) controls, again with more severely-impaired patients showing greater improvement than mildly-impaired patients.

A variety of other interventions have been studied for the treatment of neglect, but the essential ingredient of these strategies includes training in visual scanning, sometimes facilitated by strategies to promote scanning to the left hemispatial field either through incorporating movement of the left arm and hand, or through visual imagery of movement of the left arm or hand when the left arm is hemiparetic.

Visual imagery has been incorporated into scanning techniques through the use of the "Lighthouse Strategy" (LHS), in which patients were trained to use the imagery of being a lighthouse, turning from side to side in order to illuminate their surroundings (Neimeier, 1998). Neimeier (1998) used this strategy to treat 16 stroke patients with left neglect. The treatment group was, on average, two months post-stroke and treatment occurred in the context of a comprehensive day treatment program (average length of stay was 25 days). Training consisted of teaching patients to use the imagery of being a lighthouse, turning from side to side in order to illuminate their surroundings. As compared to a matched control group, the treatment group demonstrated significant improvement in overall attention on a functional task as measured by a facility rating scale and the reports of family and caregivers. These findings were supported by a follow-up study of 19 patients with visual neglect. Following treatment, patients demonstrated significant functional improvements in route finding, walking or wheelchair negotiation, and problem-solving skills (Neimeier, 2001).

In addition to visual scanning strategies, recent authors have studied various limb activation strategies in the treatment of hemispatial neglect. In these, patients are taught to move or simply attend to the affected limb prior to or during a spatial activity. These strategies are based on the finding that neglect is a lateralized attention deficit, and that motor responses on the side contralateral to the lesion increase activation of the damaged hemisphere, thereby causing change in lateralized attention (Brunila et al., 2002). Additionally, these strategies may arouse premotor circuits of the damaged hemisphere which, in turn, arouse the sensory cells associated with them, ultimately leading to perceptual enhancement of the stimuli in the neglected field (Robertson & North, 1993). In addition, it is believed that even the preparation of a motor plan, either real or imagined, serves to facilitate the perception of objects in the neglected area of space.

There are three different evidence-based limb activation strategies, including spatio-motor strategies, imagined limb activation, and visuo-spatio-motor strategies. Building on Diller and associates' earlier work on spatial reconditioning, Wiart et al. (1997) used a visuo-spatio-motor strategy called "Bon Saint Come" method to treat patients with visual neglect. Twenty-two participants, all less than three months following a stroke, were randomly assigned to either an experimental group ($n = 11$) or a control group ($n = 11$). Both groups received traditional rehabilitation, while the treatment group received an additional one hour of training combining the use of visual scanning, trunk rotation, and proprioceptive (dummy) feedback for 20 days. The treatment group demonstrated significantly greater improvements in scores on the Functional Independence Measure (FIM) and on a battery of tests for neglect as compared to the control group. However, the extent to which limb activation techniques can lead to permanent changes in neglect, as compared to only a temporary reduction in its effects during the activation itself, remains to be determined.

5.5 Visual Scanning Training

The philosophy of the use of training tasks (primarily visual cancellation tasks) for treating hemi-inattention is described in Diller and Weinberg (1977). In using a visual cancellation task that is sensitive to disturbances in visual attention, several features influence the individual's task response. Before commenting on these features, important aspects of hemi-inattention should be noted: neglect in individuals with right cerebral brain damage may be thought of as a response style in which the individual ignores or minimizes space on the left. A visual cancellation task has spatial features sensitive to this response style and thus can serve as a diagnostic tool. In turn, modifications of visual cancellation task conditions can have profound effects on improving the individual's performance and allow for its use as a training task. The following principles (see section 5.5.a below) are offered in the conceptualization of visual tasks; by using these principles to alter task demands, the training task will provide inherently greater or less structure, making task completion less or more challenging, respectively. As with all training, tasks are designed to provide greater structure earlier in training and for individuals with greater impairment. Task structure is reduced (and hopefully structure is internalized) as learning proceeds.

5.5.a Principles of Visual Scanning Training

1) **Locus of the Stimulus:** Stimuli on the left side of space are more likely to be omitted than stimuli on the right side of space.

2) **Anchoring:** When individuals are given either verbal or visual cues to begin each line at the extreme left side of the page to indicate the starting position, improvement is noted. Individuals with RBD are more influenced by anchoring on the left side of space than on the right side of space. Both types of anchoring are superior to free-style performance.

3) **Pacing:** Once the individual's orientation is anchored, there is still a tendency for rapid drifting towards targets on the right side of the page. The patient can

slow down performance to an even pace simply by reciting the targets aloud. This activity automatically harnesses the performance speed.

4) **Density:** Errors tend to occur when targets are closer to each other. It is possible to reduce errors by increasing distance between targets. An increase in font size of the visual array is another way of addressing this principle.

5) **Information Load:** Stimulus complexity increases task demands. Visual search for two targets is more difficult than visual search for a single target. Conditional target cancellation is also more difficult (e.g., cross out all the "8s," but underline the "5s."

6) **Performance Prediction and Feedback:** Asking the individual to predict performance results, as well as providing feedback on performance, are both methods of incorporating awareness into the task performance process.

5.5.b Assessment of Visual Scanning

Assessment of visual scanning for the Diller et al. (1980) protocol utilizes forms 5-1 and 5-2 provided below. The first scanning task (5-1) requires the patient to scan for a single letter "H," and the second (5-2) requires the patient to scan for two target letters, "C" and "E," simultaneously. The following instructions are provided for the one- and two-target components of the Diller-Weinberg Visual Cancellation Test.

Form 5-1 Cancel "H"

Description: An 8" X 11½" sheet of paper containing six lines of 52 letters per line. The stimulus letter "H" is scattered randomly throughout the task (105 occurrences).

Introduction: Examiner points to the middle of the top line and asks the patient to identify five or six letters. If correct, then proceed: "I want you to put a line through (cross out) every "H" that you see, without skipping any. When you are done, put your pencil down."

Scoring: Find the total number of omissions, number of commissions, and time of testing. Divide the page into thirds and determine the number of errors on each third of the page.

Form 5-2 Cancel "C" and "E"

Description: An 8" X 11½" sheet of paper containing six lines of 52 letters per line. The stimulus letters "C" and "E" are scattered randomly throughout the task (105 occurrences).

Instruction: Examiner points to the middle of the top line and asks the patient to identify five or six letters. If correct, then proceed: "I want you to put a line through (cross out) every "C" and "E" that you see, without skipping any. When you are done, put your pencil down."

Scoring: Find the total number of omissions, number of commissions, and time of testing. Divide the page into thirds and determine the number of errors on each third of the page.

5.5.c Step in Systematic and Orderly Scanning Training

These investigators (Diller et al., 1980) established very clear procedures for visual scanning training using Forms 5-3 and 5-4, which are provided on pages 99 and 100.

1) **Establish patient understanding of problem:** This training improves basic abilities and prepares the patient for training in reading. Difficulties with impulsivity are also addressed. The trainer should try to relate this training to any reading difficulties the patient may have reported.

2) **Gather and prepare materials:** Materials include two forms of cancellation tasks: single and double stimuli. Each form is an 8 ½" by 11" sheet of paper containing 312 numbers (ranging from one to nine) divided into six lines, each line having 52 stimuli. The target stimuli are randomly distributed along each line. The forms correspond to cancellation of "8," "3," & "5" on the scanning training Forms 5-3 and 5-4 (Weinberg et al., 1977). All cancellation sheets are taped on a flat surface in front of the patient. If the patient wears glasses, make sure they are clean and patient is wearing them.

3) **Training in Single Stimulus Visual Cancellation:**
   a) A vertical line is drawn on the left margin of the cancellation form by the trainer to *anchor* the left field for the patient. If needed, numbers are placed to the left and right of each line of the form to provide additional anchoring.

   b) The patient is asked to look at the anchor line at the top left margin of the page and then find the number "1" beside the anchor line.

   c) Ask the patient to scan from left to right along the first line (line #1), reading all the numbers *aloud* and crossing out every "8" along the way.

   d) The trainer should observe the patient's behavior carefully. The patient is corrected is he/she skips any "8s" in cancellation, or misreads/omits numbers while reading.

   e) When the patient has finished the cancellations on the first line, the trainer instructs the patient to scan to the left, to find the anchor line, and to use the sequential numbering of the lines in order to find the beginning of the next line. The patient may use the previously cancelled line as a *visual* guide in getting back to the beginning of the line, but actual tracing (i.e., with a pencil) of the line back to the left is discouraged.

   f) As the patient's performance improves, the number of cues can be systematically decreased:

   - Remove sequential numbers from right margin, keep anchor line and sequential numbers on the left margin, and continue to have patient read numbers aloud.

   - Remove sequential numbers from the left, but keep anchor line. Have the patient read numbers aloud.

   - Have patient perform cancellation task silently, but instruct patient to verbalize numbers to self.

   - Remove anchor line on left.

   - Gradually increase patient's speed without loss of accuracy.

   g) As cueing decreases, the patient should be given direct feedback on his/her performance. This can be done initially by circling the patient's errors, and then gradually letting the patient find his/her own errors on work completed.

   h) As training continues, or if patient shows significant unawareness, the patient should be encouraged to predict his/her performance on the Single Stimulus Visual Cancellation Task. Have the patient compare predicted with actual performance, as well as discuss the reasons for any discrepancy, in order to increase awareness of the visual difficulty.

4) **Criteria for Performance — Single Stimulus Visual Cancellation:**
   a) For the mildly impaired patient: The patient must be able to complete six lines of Single Stimulus Visual Cancellation with less than four errors scattered throughout the form.

b) For the markedly impaired patient: The patient must make one-third or less as many errors as on Diller-Weinberg Visual Cancellation Test "H" pre-test, and errors should not be concentrated on the left side of the page.

5) Training in Double Stimuli Visual Cancellation:

a) Training in double-stimuli visual cancellation follows the same procedures as in the single form (see above). This training is introduced when the patient has comfortably mastered the single stimuli cancellation task with a minimum of cueing.

b) Instruct the patient to scan from left to right along each line, crossing out every "3" and "5" seen.

c) The hierarchy of cueing (i.e., numbering lines, anchoring, verbalization, etc.), and the removal of cues, are the same as in the single stimulus visual cancellation task condition.

6) Criteria for Performance – Double Stimuli Visual Cancellation:

a) For the mildly impaired patient: The patient must be able to complete six lines of Double Stimuli Visual Cancellation with less than four errors scattered throughout the form.

b) For the markedly impaired patient: The patient must make one-third or less as many errors as on the Diller-Weinberg Visual Cancellation "C & E" pre-test, and errors should not be concentrated on the left side of the page.

5.5.d Computerized Visual Scanning Training

Pizzamiglio et al. (1992) established the following procedures as part of a broader protocol for the treatment of visual neglect. Although not recommended as a stand alone treatment, computer-based scanning tasks may be used in conjunction with paper and pencil cancellation tasks.

1) Stimuli should be projected over a large visual field (e.g., 96" horizontally by 18" vertically). The field should consist of four rows, each row allowing for stimuli to be presented in 12 different positions. Each position should be separated by 6.9" horizontally and 2.9" vertically.

2) The patient is seated approximately three feet from the screen. Single digits (size 2.3" x 1.7") are randomly presented one at a time in one of 48 positions. In each trial, each digit has an equal chance of being presented. The patient is asked to name the digit presented and press a button as quickly as possible after seeing it.

3) In each 30-minute training session, the patient is shown 20 sequences each consisting of approximately 20 digits.

4) Initially, digit sequences are presented from right to left. Early in training stimulus presentation is also preceded by a warning signal, such as a flashing bar under the target accompanied by both verbal and tactile cues from the therapist.

5) As training continues, digits are also gradually presented more towards the left visual field, so that by the end of training sequences are presented in random alternating fashion between left and right positions.

6) As the patient's performance improves, the number of cues can be decreased by removing the tactile cues, the verbal cues, and/or the warning signal.

5.5.e Visual Scanning Training for Reading and Copying Prose

Hemispatial neglect can, of course, affect reading, often referred to as neglect dyslexia. Both Diller et al. (1980) and Pizzamiglio et al. (1992) have developed training programs for the treatment of reading and copying disorders. The following procedures are based on these protocols.

1) Reading

a) **Establish patient understanding of problem:** Visual scanning difficulties can affect a patient's ability to read. This training is aimed at helping the patient compensate for neglecting the left side of pages and the beginning of words, as well as skipping lines while reading. Application to daily activities should be discussed.

b) **Materials:** Printed materials taken from the large-print and regular-print newspaper may be used for training. The large-print and regular-print *Reader's Digest* are also good sources.

c) **Training preliminaries:** Selected paragraphs of various length and content are used for training. Selected readings are placed directly in front of the patient to read.

d) **Training reading skills:**

1) Start with large-type single sentences and newspaper or magazine titles with simple, realistic content. Progress to a four-line paragraph and gradually increase the length to 10- and 15-line reading passages. Table 5-1 provides sample four-line reading stimulus material. The trainer places a red anchor line on the left, and sequential numbers on the left and right margins of each passage. The patient is asked to read the paragraph aloud, starting with line #1, and to look first for the anchor line and the sequential numbers before reading each line.

2) Begin with the minimum additional cues the patient needs to accurately read the material. Cues can be tactile (e.g., tapping the neglected shoulder), or verbal (e.g., "Remember to look carefully on your left.")

3) The trainer should observe the patient's behavior carefully and should not permit the patient to misread words, skip lines, or move the paragraph into the right visual field. Head movements are encouraged.

4) Patients may experience difficulty in locating the next line to read. If this occurs, maximum cueing should be instituted. Table 5-1 provides the sequence of cues that should be utilized. The patient is then instructed to scan to the left until he/she finds the anchor line and the sequential numbering of the lines.

5) As the patient's performance improves, the length and complexity of the reading passages can be gradually increased, while cues are systematically decreased in the following way:

- Remove sequential numbers from right margin, but keep anchor line and sequential numbers on the left margin. Have the patient read aloud.

- Remove sequential numbers from left margin, but keep anchor line. Have the patient read aloud.

- Remove anchor line on left. Have the patient read aloud.

- Transfer from large-print text to regular-size text and follow same hierarchy of cueing as needed for accurate patient performance.

- Have the patient read in silence and ask questions about the content.

- Increase the length of the passage to be read in silence.

Table 5-1 Stimulus Material and Sequence of Cueing for Four Levels of Reading Training in Neglect Dyslexia

Levels	Sequence of Cuing	Stimulus Material	Task Demand
Level 1	a) A vertical anchoring line on left side. b) Sequential numbering on left and right margins.	1- The Treasury Secretary is not now a -1 2- member of the National Security Council -2 3- but is occasionally invited to participate -3 4- in its deliberations. -4	Patient is asked to look at the anchoring line, and the number at beginning and end of lines. S/He uses vertical line to find beginning of paragraph, and uses numbers not to skip lines.
Level 2	a) A vertical anchoring line on left side. b) Sequential numbering on left margin only.	1- A growth of 6 percent in the nation's 2- output of goods and services next year 3- would be higher than what is now being 4- forecast by most economists. In the third	Patient uses only anchoring line and number at the beginning of paragraph.
Level 3	A vertical anchoring line on the left side.	Among the subjects discussed in the series of meetings, most of them an hour long, were foreign policy, international economics, government reorganization,	Patient uses only the anchoring line.
Level 4	No cues provided.	At meetings with the Senate Foreign Relations and House International Relations Committees, Mr. Obama said that he would cooperate and consult closely	Patient reads and/or copies without any cuing provided.

Form 5-1 Diller-Weinburg Visual Cancellation Test — Single Stimuli

H

B H D F C H C F H G I H C H I H B D A H C F B H D E H D A F H I C H F H B A F H E H F H C B D H F G H E

H E G H F E H D H F H C B F H A D H C E H I H G D H C E B H E G H I H C H E H F C I H E B H G F D H B E

H B H A E H B H C F A H F H G H C G D H C B A H G D E H C B E H D G H D A F H B I F H E B H D H E H G

H D G A H C H F B H A F H E B F H C D H F H G E H B H D H F A C H C H F D I H C B I H B H A C H D H F B

E H B H G B I H C E H A F H I H E B H G F B H F A H E B G H G F E H D B H B H C F H A D C H E I H F H G

H D C B H E D G H A D F H B H I G E H G H D E H C G H D H E B A H F B H C D A H G B H C H D F H C A I H

Form 5-2 Diller-Weinburg Visual Cancellation Test—Double Stimuli

C E

B E I F H E H F E G I C H E I C B D A C H F B E D A C D A F C I H C F E B A F E A C F C H B D C F G H E

C A H F A C D C F E H B F C A D E H A E I E G D E G H B C A G C I E H C I E F H I C D B C G F D E B A

E B C A F C B E H F A E F E G C H G D E H B A E G D A C H E B A E D G C D A F C B I F E A D C B E A C G

C D G A C H E F B C A F E A B F C H D E F C G A C B E D C F A H E H E F D I C H B I E B C A H C D E F B

A C B C G B I E H A C A F C I C A B E G F B E F A E A B G C F A C D B E B C H F E A D H C A D E F E G

E D H B C A D G E A D F E B E I G A C G E D C A B A E F B C H D A C G B E H C D H E H A I E

Form 5-3 Diller-Weinburg Visual Cancellation Training Sheet — Single Stimuli

8

```
2 8 4 6 3 8 3 6 8 7 9 8 3 8 9 8 2 4 1 8 3 6 2 8 4 5 8 4 1 6 8 9 3 8 6 8 2 1 6 8 5 8 6 8 3 2 4 8 6 7 8 5
8 5 7 8 6 5 8 4 8 6 8 3 2 6 8 1 4 8 2 4 8 5 7 4 8 7 5 2 8 5 7 8 9 8 3 8 5 8 5 3 9 8 6 3 5 2 8 7 6 4 8 2 5
8 2 8 1 5 8 2 8 3 6 1 8 6 8 7 8 3 7 4 8 3 2 1 8 7 4 5 8 3 8 2 5 8 4 7 8 4 1 6 8 2 9 6 8 5 2 8 4 8 5 8 7
8 4 7 1 8 3 8 6 2 8 1 6 8 5 2 6 8 8 4 8 6 8 7 5 8 2 8 4 8 6 1 8 8 6 4 9 8 3 8 6 4 9 8 3 2 9 8 2 8 1 3 8 4 8 6 2
5 8 2 7 2 9 8 3 5 8 1 6 8 9 8 5 9 8 5 2 8 6 1 8 5 2 7 8 4 2 8 2 8 6 3 8 1 4 3 8 2 8 3 6 8 1 4 3 8 5 9 8 6 8 7
8 4 3 2 8 5 4 7 8 1 4 6 8 2 8 9 7 5 8 7 8 4 5 8 3 7 8 4 8 5 2 1 8 6 2 8 7 2 8 3 4 1 8 7 2 8 3 4 6 8 3 1 9 8
```

Form 5-4 Diller-Weinburg Visual Cancellation Training Sheet — Double Stimuli

3 5

2 5 9 6 8 5 7 9 3 8 5 4 1 3 6 2 5 4 1 3 4 1 6 3 9 8 3 6 5 2 1 6 5 1 3 6 3 8 2 4 3 6 7 8 5

3 1 8 5 6 1 3 4 3 6 8 2 6 3 1 4 5 8 1 5 9 5 7 4 5 7 8 2 3 1 7 3 9 5 8 3 9 4 2 3 7 6 4 5 2 1

5 2 3 1 6 3 2 5 8 6 1 5 6 5 7 3 8 7 4 5 8 2 1 5 7 4 1 3 8 5 2 1 5 4 7 3 4 1 6 3 2 9 6 5 1 4 3 2 5 1 3 7

3 4 7 1 3 8 5 6 2 3 1 6 5 1 2 6 3 8 4 5 6 3 7 1 3 2 5 4 3 6 1 8 5 8 5 6 4 9 3 8 2 9 5 6 2

1 3 2 3 7 2 9 5 8 1 3 1 6 3 9 3 1 2 5 7 6 2 5 6 1 5 1 2 7 3 7 6 1 3 4 2 5 2 3 8 6 5 1 4 8 3 1 9 5 6 5 7

5 4 8 2 3 1 4 7 5 1 4 6 5 2 5 9 7 1 3 7 5 4 1 3 8 7 5 4 3 1 2 5 6 2 3 8 4 1 3 7 2 5 8 3 4 6 5 8 1 9 5

2) **Copying**

    a) **Establish patient understanding of problem:** This training aims at helping the patient with the mechanics of copying. Since this is a rather complex task (i.e., involving horizontal and vertical scanning, reading, and writing), it is introduced after the patient has become fairly proficient with cancellations tasks and reading.

    b) **Materials:** For copying prose, the materials are the same as for reading, plus a lined blank sheet of paper. For the line drawings, the materials include pairs of side-by-side dot matrices ranging from 4-20 dots each. In the left matrices, some dots are connected by solid lines.

    c) **Training preliminaries:** Same as for reading.

    d) **Training copying skills:**

        1) Copying Prose (Diller et al., 1980; Pizzamiglio et. al, 1992)

- Start with large-type single sentences and newspaper or magazine titles to copy. Progress to a five-line paragraph, and gradually increase to 10- and 15-line passages. Form 5-5 provides a sample stimulus of prose for copying. The trainer begins with the minimum cues the patient needs for accuracy in copying. An anchor on the left margin, and sequential numbering of right and left margins of the passage, plus an anchor and similar numbering on the lined blank sheet of paper to be used for copying, may be required, depending upon the impairment level of the patient.

- Instruct the patient to copy the text exactly as he/she sees it (including punctuation, capitals, etc.). Have the patient start by copying the words one-at-a-time and line-by-line rather than grouping the words into phrases. Then instruct the patient to scan the passage from left to right, to find the word to be copied, and to begin copying next to appropriate anchors on the lined blank sheet of paper. In addition to a red visual anchor line, tactile and/ or verbal cues may be necessary to facilitate performance.

- Initially, verbalization of words and location of the word in the passage should be encouraged. Words eventually can be grouped into dyads for scanning and then copying. Verbalization should then be phased out gradually, and the patient encouraged to perform the task in silence.

- As the patient's ability to copy gradually improves, cues can be systematically decreased as follows:

    › Progressively remove tactile and verbal cues.

    › Remove sequential numbers from right margin of passage and paper on which passage is to be copied. Have the patient read words to be copied aloud.

    › Remove sequential numbers from left margin of passage and paper, but keep anchor lines on left. Continue to have the patient read the words to be copied aloud. At this point, patient can be instructed to copy passage in a continuous flow, rather than line-by-line.

    › Remove left anchor line from passage and blank paper; continue to have the patient read the words to be copied aloud.

> Encourage patient to begin grouping words to be copied together, and continue to have patient read words to be copied aloud. Offer cueing as needed for accurate performance.

> Have the patient perform copying task in silence and gradually increase the length of the passage.

> Transfer from large-print text to regular-size print, and follow the above hierarchy of cues as needed for maintaining accuracy.

2) Copying Line Drawings (Pizzamiglio, 1992)

- The patient is presented a pair of four dot matrices; in the left matrix two dots are connected with a solid line. The patient is asked to copy this line drawing on the right matrix. A small circle indicates the point from which the patient must start their copy.

- The cueing procedure is similar to that used for copying prose.

- Once the patient is able to copy the four dot matrices accurately, gradually increase the number of dots per matrix up to 20.

5.5.f Visual Scanning for Describing Pictures

The following instructions are based upon visual scanning training procedures from Pizzamiglio et al. (1992). This picture description activity is included as part of a broader protocol including visual scanning for numbers in a large visual field, reading and copying training, and copying of line drawings.

a) **Materials:** Black and white pictures of simple figures and realistic scenes with a dimension of 30-42cm.

b) **Training in Figure Description:**

1) Start with simple figures and drawings. The patient is asked to describe all of the essential features depicted in the presented drawing or scene.

2) When stimuli are omitted, verbal cues are provided to aid performance. Cues may be generic (e.g., "Do you see anything else in this picture?"), or they may be specific with the aim or directing the patient's attention to missing elements.

Form 5-5   Sample Stimulus Material for Copying

1- Up in Kentville, Nova Scotia, Walter   -1
2- Wood, said to be the world's oldest Boy   -2
3- Scout, recently celebrated his 103rd -3
4- birthday. Mr. Wood, who emigrated to   -4
5- Nova Scotia from Britain when he was   -5
6- 20 years old, received Scouting's high-   -6
7- est honor, the Silver Wolf Medal, in   -7
8- 1975. Did he expect to celebrate his   -8
9- 104th birthday? Mr. Wood's reply was   -9
10- to note the Boy Scout motto, "Be pre-   -10
11- pared."   -11

1-	-1
2-	-2
3-	-3
4-	-4
5-	-5
6-	-6
7-	-7
8-	-8
9-	-9
10-	-10
11-	-11

Figure: Copying Task Showing Maximum Cuing Provided on Paragraph to be Copied and "Blank Page" Upon Which to Copy

5.6 Visual Imagery Training: Lighthouse Strategy

Niemeier (1998) and Niemeier et al., (2001) described the "Lighthouse Strategy" used in the treatment of hemispatial neglect. The following steps are to be utilized for training.

1) When engaging in a task that requires visual attention, the patient is asked to imagine that they are a lighthouse and is shown a picture of one, if available. The therapist places a picture of a lighthouse in the farthest aspect of the left hemispatial field to which the patient can direct their visual attention. The patient is then asked to imagine that his/her eyes are like the lights inside the top of the lighthouse, sweeping all the way to the left and right of the horizon to guide the ships at sea to safety.

2) The therapist might ask, "What would happen if the lighthouse lit only on the right side of the ocean and horizon?" After the patient responds, the therapist says, "Let's try this," and introduces a simple computer-assisted, paper and pencil task, or table-top activity requiring full scanning of left and right hemispatial fields to be performed correctly.

3) The width of the visual stimuli to be scanned should be noted and controlled so as to challenge the patient, but at the same time ensure that the patient can succeed on some trials. If the therapist is using a computer, it may be important to use a large monitor that requires scanning to the outer edges of the visual field (Webster et al., 2001).

4) When the patient misses some of the stimuli, he or she is told, "Look, you missed these on the left (or right). Let's try that again, but this time pretend you are that lighthouse and turn your head from side to side to allow your eyes to sweep left and right like the light in the top of a lighthouse." The therapist provides a demonstration of the proper degree and rate of head turning, and the patient is also shown how to line up their chin first with the top of their right, and then the top of their left shoulder.

5) After completing the table-top activity, the patient is asked to count or locate items in the room on their right and left sides. Verbal and tactile cues are provided as needed to facilitate performance.

6) Initial training sessions focus on visually scanning paper-and-pencil, computer-assisted visual or simple functional tasks. With progress, subsequent training sessions incorporate ambulation or wheelchair negotiation tasks, and the patient is asked to identify target visual stimuli posted throughout the environment, or with periodic requests for the patient to locate people or objects on both sides. Physical cues such as lightly tapping the neglected shoulder can be used as well as verbal cues, both of which can be faded as the patient improves his or her ability to apply the strategy independently to training tasks.

5.6.a Activities for Training in Visual Scanning and the Use of the Lighthouse Strategy

Acquisition and Application Stages:

- Attention Process Training — large and small shape, number and letter cancellation tasks
- Computer-based scanning and tracking programs
- Computer-based reading programs
- Other simple reading materials
- Paper and pencil tasks (drawing, copying, coloring, writing etc.)

- Counting or locating pictures or objects spread out on a table
- Locating or counting objects or people within the treatment room
- Drawing and picture descriptions

Application and Adaptation Stages:

- Magazines, newspapers, novels, and textbooks
- Internet navigation tasks
- Locating keys on computer keyboard, icons on computer desktop, or tabs on the left side of program menus, web pages, etc.
- Computer-based reading fluency programs
- Following recipe instructions
- Cooking and shopping
- Locating items in a cluttered drawer or kitchen
- Locating, counting and/or navigating around people or objects during ambulation or wheelchair navigation
- Map reading and/or locating items on a map
- Locating treatment rooms or other target locations on the left side of the hallway while navigating facility
- Responding to targets on left side of screen during driving simulation task, or while playing video games
- Looking both ways before safely crossing the street

5.7 Limb Activation Strategies

5.7.a Spatio-Motor Strategies

Spatio-motor strategies encourage the patient to move their left hand, arm, or shoulder as much as possible immediately before or during visual training tasks. Some techniques have involved asking the patient to tap the table as many times as possible with the left hand (Wilson et al., 2000), or asking the patient to clench and open their left hand repeatedly, or if unable to do that, to simply lift their shoulder on the left, during the performance of the task (Brunila et al., 2002; Worthington, 1996).

5.7.b Visuo-Spatio-Motor Strategies

Visuo-spatio-motor strategies utilize both scanning and limb activation simultaneously. Research has demonstrated the success of this strategy in treating some cases of hemispatial neglect (Samuel et al., 2000; Worthington, 1996). It should be noted that this approach reflects a combination of the visual scanning strategy of "anchoring" and visuo-motor cueing.

1) During a reading task (or any visual scanning task) the patient is asked to: (a) place their left hand at the margin of the visual stimulus they are to visually scan; (b) look at their left hand; and (c) scan across the page until they complete the scanning task. The training involves teaching the patient to "scan to your hand."

2) In subsequent sessions, the patient can be taught to use this phrase as a means of cueing themselves to attend to the left side while performing reading or scanning tasks. Additionally, it is also recommended that the patient move his/her left arm before and during the scanning activity, if possible.

3) Movements that are most helpful are those that visually cue the patient to the left side of space (visuo-spatio-motor cueing) while activating the left limb at the

same time. Patients can be trained to move their left arm and to look at it when they unable to find the target of an exercise. If a patient fails to explore the left hemispatial field spontaneously, they should be cued to move their left arm and try again.

A similar technique, called the "Bon Saint Come" method (Wiart et al., 1997), involves the combined use of a biofeedback device and voluntary trunk rotation to improve performance on tasks requiring visual scanning. The following steps are involved in training.

1) The patient is taught how to use a device to search for lights on a lightboard. Initially, the patient is seated, and is wearing a vest that has a vertical metal bar attached to it. The pointer of the bar projects forward horizontally just above the apex of their head. In order to touch a target, the patient needs to rotate their trunk to move the device.

2) During the first sessions, a spotlight is used to cue visual fixation to the left side of the board. The patient is then required to detect visual and/or auditory signals and slowly move from the left to right side to locate and touch the target with the pointer. If the patient succeeds, the same visual and auditory signals are emitted, providing positive feedback. Incorrect responses provoke no response, and the patient has to try again.

3) As the patient's trunk control improves, they do the same exercises from a standing position. As treatment progresses, sessions can increase in duration from 15 minutes building up to an hour, according to the patient's capabilities.

4) Once the patient is able to successfully use the strategy, the technique can be adapted to other activities, without the need for the machine.

As is always the case, systematic data collection in the rehabilitation of neglect is very important. The therapist is encouraged to use the forms in Appendix B for data collection and graph these data, not only to determine if the rehabilitation strategies being utilized are resulting in progress, but for the patient and interested others to have feedback about progress. Actively engaging the patient in data collection also promotes the meaningfulness and relevance of rehabilitation.

5.7.c Activities for Training in the use of Spatio-Motor and Visuo-Spatio-Motor Strategies:

- Large and small shape, number and letter cancellation tasks using a boundary line as well as the hand as visual anchors

- Reading materials (magazines, novels, newspapers, maps, textbooks), again using the hand and a boundary line as visual anchors

- Locating keys on computer keyboard

- Paper and pencil tasks (drawing, copying, coloring, writing)

- Any activity of daily living (grooming, eating, dressing)

- Cooking

- Functional physical activities (transfers, wheelchair negotiation, ambulation)

- Scanning for particular road signs when a passenger in a car

5.7.d Imagined Limb Activation

When hemiparesis is so dense that no active movement is possible, imagined limb activation can be used. McCarthy et al., (2002) describe a procedure in which patients are asked only to visualize moving the left arm. In this procedure, the therapist directs the patient to perform a number of upper extremity movements with the unaffected right arm.

These include: (1) bending the arm at the elbow; (2) clenching the fist; (3) unclenching the fist; (4) stretching out the arm; (5) stretching out the fingers; (6) wiggling the fingers; and (7) pinching the fingers and thumb together. This sequence is then repeated with the same arm. Following this, the patient is asked to imagine performing these tasks, first with the right arm, and then with the affected left arm. Then, at various points during the completion of a task, the patient is again asked to imagine moving the left arm in the same set of movements.

One potential problem with this technique can be its level of difficulty. Imagining oneself engaging in even a simple motor activity can be difficult, particularly for those with additional impairments in body schema, sustained attention, working memory, or executive functioning. Also, the determination of whether the utilization of this technique is helpful must be based on the patient's performance on visual scanning, as it is obviously not possible for the therapist to know if the patient is able to imagine movement, other than based on their self-report. For these reasons, it is important for therapists to carefully question their patients during and after using this technique: "Were you able to imagine moving your arm? On a scale of 1-10, where 10 is perfect success, how did you do? Was there anything about the task that caused problems for you?"

5.8 Strategic and Tactical Goal Writing for the Rehabilitation of Hemispatial Neglect

PATIENT SR: Goals for Training in the use of the Lighthouse Strategy

Long-Term Strategic Goal:

Ms. SR will remember and use the Lighthouse Strategy to compensate for her left hemispatial neglect during training tasks.

Monthly Strategic Treatment Goal:

Initiate/Continue _____ stage (e.g., acquisition, application) of Lighthouse Strategy training.

Short-Term Tactical Treatment Goals:

STGa: Ms. SR will demonstrate effective use of the Lighthouse Strategy during training tasks with maximum verbal, visual, and tactile cues.

STGb: Ms. SR will perform large shape cancellation tasks (using a left side boundary marker) with 75% accuracy and maximum verbal cues to use the Lighthouse Strategy.

STGc: Ms. SR will perform small shape cancellation tasks (using a boundary marker) with fewer than two left side errors and moderate verbal cues to use the lighthouse strategy.

STGd: Ms. SR will scan for and locate keys on a computer keyboard with 90% accuracy and minimum verbal cues to use the Lighthouse Strategy.

STGe: Ms. SR will scan for and locate icons on the left side of computer screen with 100% accuracy and intermittent cues to use the Lighthouse Strategy.

STGf: Ms. SR will independently track and respond to visual stimulus moving left to right at slow speed on computer screen with 90% accuracy.

STGg: Ms. SR will independently scan for, and locate visual stimulus, presented to left visual field in time decreased by 5% of baseline.

Long-Term Strategic Goal:

Ms. SR will effectively use the Lighthouse Strategy to compensate for her left hemispatial neglect during daily functional activities.

Monthly Strategic Treatment Goal:

Initiate/Continue adaptation stage of Lighthouse Strategy training.

Short-Term Tactical Treatment Goals:

STGa: Ms. SR will scan for and locate items on left side of treatment room on 7/10 trials with moderate verbal cues to use the Lighthouse Strategy.

STGb: Ms. SR will attend to speaker on left side of treatment room on 9/10 trials with minimum verbal and tactile cues.

STGc: Ms. SR will scan for and locate target objects on the left side of table during cooking activity with 90% accuracy and intermittent verbal cues to use the Lighthouse Strategy.

STGd: Ms. SR will independently use the Lighthouse Strategy to scan for and locate 9/10 target items on left side of supermarket shelf.

STGe: Ms. SR will navigate around 100% of obstacles on her neglected side during ambulation activities with intermittent cues to use the Lighthouse Strategy.

STGf: Ms. SR will independently use the Lighthouse Strategy to scan for oncoming traffic in both directions during outdoor ambulation task on 5/5 trials.

STGg: Ms. SR will independently scan for and locate tabs on left side of web page during internet training activity with 100% accuracy.

STGh: Ms. SR will independently use the Lighthouse Strategy to locate target objects on her neglected side during cooking task in time decreased by 5% of baseline.

STGi: Ms. SR will perform reading fluency task on computer in time decreased by 10% of baseline.

PATIENT TM: Goals for Training in the use of Spatio-Motor or Imagined Limb Activation Strategies

Long-Term Strategic Goal:

Mr. TM will independently remember and use spatio-motor (or imagined limb activation) strategies to improve his awareness of, and attention to, his neglected side during daily functional activities.

Monthly Strategic Treatment Goal:

Initiate/Continue _____ stage (e.g., acquisition, application, adaptation) of Spatio-motor and/or Imagined Limb Activation Strategies

Short-Term Tactical Treatment Goals:

STGa: Mr. TM will perform left upper extremity exercises prior to initiating visual scanning tasks with maximum verbal, visual, and tactile cues.

STGb: Mr. TM will perform imagined limb activation exercises prior to engaging in bed to wheelchair transfer task with maximum verbal, visual, and tactile cues.

STGc: Mr. TM will continually engage in hand tapping exercise with his left hand while performing reading task with moderate verbal cues.

STGd: Mr. TM will independently initiate use of visualization strategy prior to performing reading task during 1/5 treatment sessions.

STGe: Mr. TM will independently initiate and perform ten left shoulder shrug exercises prior to engaging in dressing task during 5/5 treatment sessions.

PATIENT BG: Goals for Training in the use of Visuo-Spatial-Motor Strategies

Long-Term Strategic Goal:

Ms. BG will effectively use visuo-spatio-motor strategies to improve her awareness of and attention to her neglected side during her daily functional activities.

Monthly Strategic Treatment Goal:

Initiate/Continue _____ stage (e.g., acquisition, application, adaptation) of visuo-spatial-motor strategy training.

Short-Term Tactical Treatment Goals:

STGa: Ms. BG will perform large shape cancellation tasks with 75% accuracy with maximum verbal, visual, and tactile cues (including using a boundary line and left hand placement as anchors).

STGb: Ms. BG will complete figure copying task with fewer than two left side omissions with moderate verbal cues, and use of a boundary marker and left hand placement as visual anchors.

STGc: Ms. BG will attend to her neglected side during ambulation task with moderate verbal and tactile cues.

STGd: Ms. BG will scan for and locate visual stimulus on the left side of cancellation tasks with 90% accuracy (using both a boundary line and left hand placement as visual anchors) and minimum verbal cues.

STGe: Ms. BG will locate food on left side of dinner plate with boundary marker, left hand placed on edge of plate and intermittent verbal cues.

STGf: Ms. BG will independently attend to her neglected left side and initiate left upper limb movement prior to performing transfer task.

STGg: Ms. BG will independently use compensatory strategies to cue herself to attend to her neglected side while performing reading task.

6. Rehabilitation of Impairments of Social Communication

6.1 Introduction

Social skills training has a long, successful history for treating the social communication deficits of individuals with psychiatric conditions and developmental disabilities. Traditional techniques of social skills training include shaping through explicit reinforcement of appropriate behaviors, role play, and audio or video feedback. These techniques have been useful in helping to increase prosocial behaviors, such as active listening, and reduce antisocial behaviors, such as interrupting (Flanagan et al., 1995).

Structured, concrete interventions that provide immediate feedback and active practice are approaches that can accommodate the cognitive impairments often experienced by individuals with TBI. However, due to deficits in social and emotional perception that are often seen in individuals with TBI, traditional approaches should be enhanced by the inclusion of explicit training in social and emotional perception. Moreover, since mood symptoms such as anxiety and depression can directly impact social functioning, interventions that incorporate psychotherapy or coping skills training may be especially important for individuals with TBI.

6.2 Impairments of Social Communication after Brain Injury

Many individuals who have sustained a TBI demonstrate a perceptible change in social behavior and reduction in social skills. These changes are often experienced as being the most impairing injury-related deficits, as poor social skills can contribute to interpersonal problems, fewer employment opportunities, reduced community integration, and feelings of isolation, depression, and reduced quality of life.

Specific deficits in social communication after TBI may include egocentricity (a tendency to focus on oneself, often to the exclusion of considering others), insensitivity to others, excessive talking, or failure to maintain appropriate social boundaries. Alternatively, some individuals may be unable to initiate social contact or maintain a social interaction. Many of these deficits are thought to be related to frontally-mediated brain systems. However, many types of cognitive impairments can contribute to difficulties in social communication. For example, a person with slowed information processing speed may have difficulty following a conversation, and consequently be unable to provide a relevant response in a timely manner. Someone with executive dysfunction and related disinhibition may have a hard time holding back from saying or doing inappropriate or impulsive things. A person with impaired memory may not recognize a person he or she met a few days prior, or may be unable to recall personally relevant information about friends or family. Impaired ability to judge or interpret emotion-related stimuli is common after TBI, and can deprive a person of the emotional cues and social feedback that would otherwise help them to guide their behavior. Emotional factors, such as reduced self-esteem, and mood disorders such as anxiety or depression, can also contribute to anti-social behavior and social withdrawal.

Successful interpersonal interaction requires both a solid repertoire of adaptive social behaviors and the ability to interpret and make use of social cues and feedback. Deficits in any of these skills can have a devastating impact on social communication. Individuals with TBI who experience repeated failures in social contexts may become socially withdrawn, and/or an individual's poor social communication may strain relationships and provide a disincentive for friends and family to maintain relationships. The treatment approaches described here can help to remediate the skills required for adaptive interpersonal communication.

6.3 BI-ISIG Recommendations for the Rehabilitation of Impairments of Social Communication

The BI-ISIG Cognitive Rehabilitation Task Force of ACRM has reviewed four high-quality (Class I) research studies that have investigated interventions for cognitive-communication deficits in individuals with TBI. These studies support the Task Force's recommendation that specific intervention for functional communication deficits, including pragmatic conversational skills, are recommended for social communication skills after TBI as a Practice Standard (Cicerone et al., 2011). Group based interventions may be considered as a Practice Option for remediation of social-communication deficits after TBI.

Group Interactive Structured Treatment (GIST): for Social Competence (Hawley & Newman, 2006, 2008), an intervention addressing the communication, cognitive, and emotional skills and behaviors necessary for successful social interaction, was found to be efficacious in reducing functional impairments in social communication and improving overall satisfaction with life (Dahlberg et al., 2007). A program that provided focused training in pragmatic communication behaviors (i.e., listening, initiating a conversation) and social perception in addition to providing individual psychotherapy, has been shown to facilitate emotional adjustment and improved adaptation in social situations (McDonald et al., 2008). Focused training in emotional perception has been shown to produce improvements in recognition of others' emotional expressions, but did not produce more general improvements in psychosocial functioning. Particular strategies for emotional perception training (namely, errorless learning and self-instructional training) are effective in helping individuals with TBI to better judge facial expressions and make social inferences (Bornhofen & McDonald, 2007; Bornhofen & McDonald, 2008).

Two general approaches to the rehabilitation of social communication impairments have been reviewed and recommended by the BI-ISIG Task Force. These include Social Skills Treatment and Treatment of Emotion Perception Deficits, which will be presented here.

6.4 A General Framework for the Rehabilitation of Impairments of Social Communication

The goal of any social communication skills treatment program is to help participants to develop skills in the following areas: communication of needs and thoughts; listening to and understanding others; using and interpreting nonverbal messages; regulation of emotions; conforming to appropriate social boundaries and rules; working with others to solve problems; and assertiveness (Hawley & Newman, 2006). Specific aspects of social behavior can be addressed, such as greetings, introducing oneself, listening, giving compliments, initiating a conversation, selecting and maintaining a topic, being assertive, and coping with disagreements (McDonald et al., 2008).

Group-based interventions are well suited to the rehabilitation of social communication impairments. Groups can provide a safe and structured social microcosm in which new behaviors can be learned, practiced, and rehearsed. Participants receive immediate feedback from other group members and from the clinical professionals who are leading the group. Group interventions for social skills address specific social skills or behaviors in a group format, and individual treatment goals are set and monitored throughout treatment. Role play, feedback through video or audio taped social interactions, and generalization of learned skills to natural settings are key components of successful group interventions. Significant others and family members are often encouraged to become involved in the treatment process by learning methods of delivering helpful feedback or assisting in the completion of homework assignments. (Hawley & Newman, 2006, 2008; Hawley & Newman, 2010; McDonald, 2008).

6.5 Group Treatment for Social Communication Deficits

The protocols for group treatment for social communication deficits were developed by Hawley & Newman (2006, 2008) and McDonald and colleagues (2008), and the following information was adapted from two workbooks: *Group Interactive Structured Treatment-GIST: for Social Competence*, Hawley and Newman, (2006, 2008), www.braininjurysocialcompetence.com and *Improving First Impressions: A Step-by-Step Social Skills Program*, McDonald et al., (2009). http://www.assbi.com.au/resources/ImprovingFirstImpressions.pdf.

6.5.a Structure

Individuals with TBI tend to function best in environments that are structured and predictable. Knowing what to expect can minimize anticipatory anxiety, reduce cognitive load, and allow individuals to prepare for upcoming tasks. Consequently, all group sessions should follow the same general structure and format. An example of a group structure:

1. Review of homework
2. Brief introduction of topic or target skill to be addressed (see below for suggested topics)
3. Guided discussion
4. Small group practice with therapist modeling and/or role play
5. Group problem-solving and feedback
6. Homework assignment

Suggested Group Topics

- Orientation and review of group; participants "tell their story"
- Key social communication skills – greetings, introductions, listening, giving compliments, turn taking, asking questions, interest in your conversational partner
- Self-assessment of communication skills and goal setting
- Starting conversations, topic selection
- Keeping conversations going and using feedback
- Being assertive, problem-solving and coping with disagreements
- Social confidence and positive self talk
- Social boundaries
- Videotaping and video review
- Conflict Resolution
- Community outing as a group

6.5.b Group Process

Group treatment provides ample opportunity for structured interaction, in-the-moment feedback, and a forum in which to test out and practice newly-learned or modified social skills. Additionally, a group provides a network of support and a source of belonging, while sending the message that participants are not alone in their challenges. Positive social reinforcement helps to build confidence and motivation for treatment. An ideal group size is four to eight participants, as this size tends to allow for the development of group interaction while preserving sufficient time for individual attention.

6.5.c Individual Goal Setting

Individual goal setting places an emphasis on self-awareness, self-monitoring, and self-assessment. Participants' unique difficulties with different aspects of social communication should be identified so that treatment can be appropriately tailored. For example, an individual who has difficulty remembering people's names might have different social challenges than a person who has difficulty staying on topic during a conversation. Initial group sessions focus on the identification and specification of specific individual goals to work on during treatment. Due to limitations in awareness of deficits commonly seen after TBI, the goal-setting process should be a collaborative effort between an individual and the clinician(s) and/or family members. It is important that goals be personally relevant to the individual participant in order to maximize their motivation for treatment. After goal selection, each individual goal is broken down into realistic and measurable steps and rated by the clinician and group participant. This helps the participant be successful in achieving each step toward the overall goal (see examples listed below). Identifying goals through self-assessment helps increase awareness, and achieving steps towards a goal may increase the participant's sense of self-efficacy and motivation for treatment.

Examples of individual goals as part of the social communication group intervention: Start the participant's current level of performance at step two (just in case there is a decrease in the goal behavior), and then determine achievable steps to meet the goal:

Goal: I will ask on-topic questions in conversations.

1. I never ask on-topic questions in conversations.
2. I ask on-topic questions in conversations once a week.
3. I ask on-topic questions in conversations three times a week.
4. I ask on-topic questions in conversations once a day.
5. I ask on-topic questions in conversations more than once a day.

Goal: I will not interrupt during a 15 minute conversation.

1. I interrupt **more than 4 times** during a 15 minute conversation.
2. I interrupt **less than 4 times** during a 15 minute conversation.
3. I interrupt **less than 2 times** during a 15 minute conversation.
4. I interrupt **only one time** during a 15 minute conversation.
5. I do **not interrupt** during a 15 minute conversation.

6.5.d Feedback

As specific social behaviors and strategies are explored and practiced throughout the group treatment, frequent opportunities for feedback from group members and clinicians can help participants to fine-tune their skills. Group leaders can model appropriate methods of delivering feedback. Feedback is particularly powerful in the middle and later sessions of group treatment, once participants have had a chance to develop rapport with one another and with group leaders. Rather than being critical or punitive (e.g., "It's inappropriate to make a comment like that."), helpful feedback is collaborative in nature and remains oriented on the communication goals being worked toward (e.g., "What cues did you notice from the woman you met?" or "I wonder how she felt about your comment?").

6.5.e Practice and Repetition

Extensive repetition of guiding principles and practice of target behaviors or strategies can facilitate learning and memory for new skills. Exercises given as "homework" can extend the practice of techniques learned in individual or group treatment settings.

6.5.f Self-Monitoring

McDonald and colleagues (2008) recommend the use of an acronym (WSTC: What am I doing? What is the best Strategy? Try it. Check it out) that can be used and practiced throughout all treatment sessions to facilitate the development of effective planning and self-monitoring skills. By fostering the ability to evaluate one's own behavior accurately, participants can become more independent in the process of monitoring and adjusting social behaviors.

6.5.g Generalization of Skills

It is important for any rehabilitation program to include opportunities for participants to practice learned strategies and skills in natural environments to enhance generalization and carryover of gains. One way to do this is by assigning homework assignments that are appropriate to an individual's skill level (e.g., "Research three places where you might meet new people, and visit one of these places this weekend." or "Ask your significant other for specific feedback on your active listening skills."). Involving friends and family in the treatment process can create multiple opportunities for participants to practice communication skills and receive feedback in their own environments. Another way to enhance generalization of skills is to include community outings in the group schedule, during which participants can practice goal-directed behaviors such as asking a stranger for directions, or socializing with group members and leaders in a naturalistic setting such as a coffee shop or restaurant. This provides an opportunity to practice communication skills while managing external stimuli, background noise, and unanticipated interruptions or events.

6.6 Treatment of Emotion Perception Deficits

Some researchers and clinicians find that certain individuals with TBI have difficulty benefitting from traditional approaches to social skills training because they lack the ability to recognize and interpret others' nonverbal cues, such as facial expressions, tone of voice, and body posture. Without these abilities, individuals will be unable to adjust their behavior in varying social contexts.

Treatment of deficits in emotional perception often focuses on specific skills, such as recognizing specific patterns of changes in facial features and facial expression, tone of voice, body posture, and movement as they relate to the nonverbal expression of emotion. Games and other exercises can be employed to allow repetitive practice of perception skills. For more information, see:
http://www.assbi.com.au/resources/ImprovingFirstImpressions.pdf.

The presentation of learning objectives is structured hierarchically, so that more basic knowledge relating to social communication is presented initially, and provides a foundation upon which subsequent skills can be learned. Early sessions might focus on general discussions that develop a knowledge base of conventional emotional contexts, identifying emotions associated with particular scenarios (e.g., giving a public speech, celebrating a birthday, losing a loved one), and discriminating between similar or co-occurring emotions (e.g., sadness and regret, anger, and disappointment). In learning and practicing emotional perception skills, cues are hierarchically organized so that participants might be asked to judge static emotional cues from line drawings, then photographs, and then in video tapes. Cues might first be presented in one modality (e.g., visual), and then with multiple modalities (e.g., visual and auditory) presented simultaneously. Finally, fine-tuning of emotional perception skills is achieved by learning to interpret situational cues: a speaker's emotional demeanor or body language, or tone of voice. In these final stages, participants learn to make social inferences about a speaker's intentions, truthfulness, or emotional state. Throughout treatment, distributed and massed practice, rehearsal of skills, and cumulative review of previously learned material are provided to enhance retention and generalization.

Two general rehabilitation techniques have been employed in the treatment of emotion perception deficits: Errorless Learning; and Self-instruction Training. The application of these techniques to the treatment of emotion perception deficits will be discussed here.

6.6.a Errorless Learning

Errorless learning can be used to help improve emotion perception skills among individuals with intact implicit memory functioning, but impaired explicit memory.

Errorless learning involves closely guided instruction with repeated rehearsal and practice of newly learned information, and participants are specifically instructed NOT to make a guess when they are unsure of an answer. For example, if an individual is asked to identify a speaker's demeanor based on their tone of voice, but is not entirely sure whether the speaker was sarcastic or friendly, the clinician would inform them of the speaker's demeanor and then re-play the audio clip.

6.6.b Self-instruction Training

Self-instruction training involves verbalization of procedural steps by participants as they complete a complex task. The acronym "WATER" is used at first by the therapist, and eventually the participant, as a structure to approach emotion discrimination tasks. (1) *W*hat am I deciding about?; (2) *W*hat do I *A*lready know about it?; (3) *T*ry out my answer; (4) *E*valuate how it went;. (5) *R*eward myself for having a go. The participant is trained to use these self guiding statements to intensify attention to discriminating emotions in a step-by-step manner, and self correct errors when they occur. For example, this technique could be used to help a participant make social inferences on the basis of dynamic emotional and situational cues. (Bornhofen & McDonald 2008).

6.7 Individual Psychotherapy and the Treatment of Impairments of Social Communication

Some group-based treatment programs are effectively supplemented with individual (one-on-one) treatment sessions with a trained clinician. The purpose of these sessions is to facilitate adjustment to living with a long-term disability, enhance coping skills, and address mood issues such as anxiety, depression, or reduced self-esteem that might be experienced. Individual sessions can also provide an important opportunity to reinforce the strategies and skills learned during group sessions, and to further individualize and tailor treatment to meet personal needs.

Cognitive behavioral therapeutic techniques, which emphasize the use of cognitive strategies and self-talk, awareness of emotional triggers and responses, recordkeeping, repetition, relaxation training, and structured assignments, are well-suited to individuals with TBI given the cognitive impairments commonly experienced by this population.

6.8 Strategic and Tactical Goal Writing in the Rehabilitation of Impairments of Social Communication

PATIENT PP: Goals for Social Skills Training

Long-Term Strategic Goal

Mrs. PP will independently employ self-monitoring strategies to effectively participate in conversations with familiar communication partners.

Monthly Strategic Treatment Goal

Initiate/Continue _____ stage (e.g. acquisition, application, adaptation) of social skills training.

Short-Term Tactical Treatment Goals

STGa: Mrs. PP will independently identify four strategies (e.g., ask a new question, pause, ask for more information….) to use during conversations for topic maintenance and equal partner talking opportunities.

STGb: Mrs. PP will demonstrate complete topic maintenance during a 3-5 minute conversation.

STGc: Mrs. PP will independently employ the use of pausing at least 2-3 times to facilitate conversational turn-taking during a 3-5 minute conversation.

STGd: Mrs. PP will initiate 2-3 novel questions during a 3-5 minute conversation to assure balanced speaking time.

STGe: Mrs. PP will precede use of a pronoun with proper reference (e.g., name of person, prior to use of "he/she") in conversation in 80% of opportunities.

STGf: Mrs. PP will identify objective use of strategies with 80% accuracy during video review of previously taped conversations.

6.9 Strategic and Tactical Goal Writing in the Rehabilitation of Impairments of Visual Emotion Perception

PATIENT CM: Goals for Visual Emotion Perception Training

Long-Term Strategic Goal:

Mr. CM will independently name the emotions represented in pictures of people.

Monthly Strategic Treatment Goal

Initiate/Continue _____ stage (e.g., acquisition, application, adaptation) of visual emotion perception training.

Short-Term Tactical Treatment Goals

STGa: Mr. CM will identify emotion of people in complex scenarios based on photographic stimuli with a choice of six text options with 90% accuracy.

STGb: Mr. CM will identify common emotions associated with specific facial expressions with 90% accuracy.

STGc: Mr. CM will independently identify emotion in people in complex scenarios based on photographic stimuli with 90% accuracy.

6.10 Example Treatment Goal and Strategies for Use with Auditory Emotion Perception

PATIENT OC: Goals for Auditory Emotion Perception Training

Long-Term Strategic Goal

Ms. OC will independently state the emotion when provided vocal tone in verbal messages in a structured clinic setting.

Monthly Strategic Treatment Goal

Initiate/Continue _____ stage (e.g., acquisition, application, adaptation) of auditory emotion perception training.

Short-Term Tactical Treatment Goals

STGa: Ms. OC will identify the emotion of spoken messages in semantically neutral sentences with exaggerated affective tone, presented without accompanying visual information, with a choice of six text options with 90% accuracy.

STGb: Ms. OC will identify the emotion of spoken messages in semantically neutral sentences with exaggerated affective tone, presented without accompanying visual information with 90% accuracy.

STGc: Ms. OC will identify two ambiguous aspects of a communication message when conflicting visual, semantic and/or affective tone are presented with 90% accuracy.

References

Alderman, N., Fry, R., & Youngson, H. (1995) Improvement of self-monitoring skills, reduction of behavior disturbance and the dysexecutive syndrome: Comparison of response cost and a new programme of self-monitoring training. *Neuropsychological Rehabilitation*, 5, 193-221.

Bornhofen, C. & McDonald, S. (2008) Treating deficits in emotion perception following traumatic brain injury. *Neuropsychological Rehabilitation*, 18:1, 22-44.

Bornhofen, C. & McDonald, S. (2008) Comparing strategies for treating emotion perception deficits in traumatic brain injury. *Journal of Head Trauma Rehabilitation*, 23:2, 103-115.

Brush, J. & Camp, C. (1998) *A Therapy Technique for Improving Memory: Spaced Retrieval*. Meyers Research Institute. http://store.myersresearch.org/thteforimmes.html.

Brunila, T., Lincoln, N., Lindell, A., Tenovuo, O., & Hamalainen, H. (2002) Experiences of combined visual training and arm activation in the rehabilitation of unilateral visual neglect: A clinical study. *Neuropsychological Rehabilitation*, 12, 27-40.

Cantor, J.B. *Executive plus: Preliminary results*. Presentation, Federal Interagency Conference on Traumatic Brain Injury, Washington, DC: 2011, June.

Cheng, S. & Man, D. (2006) Management of impaired self-awareness in persons with traumatic brain injury. *Brain Injury*, 20, 621-628.

Cicerone, K. (2002) Remediation of working attention in mild traumatic brain injury. *Brain Injury*, 16, 185-195.

Cicerone, K., Dahlberg, C., Kalmar, K., Langenbahn, D., Malec, J., Bergquist, T. et al. (2000) Evidence-based cognitive rehabilitation: Recommendations for clinical practice. *Archives of Physical Medicine and Rehabilitation*, 81, 1596-1615.

Cicerone, K.D., Dahlberg, M.A., Malec, J.F., Langenbahn, D.M., Felicetti, T., Kneipp, S., Ellmo, W., Kalmar, K., Giacino, J.T., Harley, J.P., Laatsch, L., Morse, P.A., & Catanese, J. (2005) Evidence-based cognitive rehabilitation: updated review of the literature from 1998 to 2002. *Archives of Physical Medicine and Rehabilitation*, 86, 1681-1692.

Cicerone, K.D., Mott T., Azulay J., Sharlow-Galella, M.A., Ellmo, W.J., Paradise, S., & Friel, J.C. (2008) A randomized controlled trial of holistic neuropsychological rehabilitation after traumatic brain injury. *Archives of Physical Medicine and Rehabilitation*, 89, 2239-2249.

Cicerone, K.D., Langenbahn, D.M., Braden, C., Malec, J.F., Kalmar, K., Fraas, M., Felicetti, T., Laatsch, L., Harley, J.P., Bergquist, T., Azulay J., Cantor, J., & Ashman, T. (2011) Evidence-based cognitive rehabilitation: updated review of the literature from 2003 through 2008. *Archives of Physical Medicine and Rehabilitation*, 9, 519-530.

Cicerone, K. & Giacino, J. (1992) Remediation of executive function deficits after traumatic brain injury. *NeuroRehabilitation*, 2, 12-22.

Cicerone, K., Mott, T., Azulay, J., & Friel, J.C. (2004) Community integration and satisfaction with functioning after intensive cognitive rehabilitation for traumatic brain injury. *Archives of Physical Medicine and Rehabilitation*, 85, 943-950.

Cicerone, K.D. & Wood, J.C. (1987) Planning disorder after closed head injury: a case study. *Archives of Physical Medicine and Rehabilitation*, 68, 111-115.

Crosson, B., Barco, P.P., Velozo, C.A., Bolesta, M., Cooper, P.V., Werts, D., & Broebeck, T.C. (1989) Awareness and compensation in postacute head injury rehabilitation. *Journal of Head Trauma Rehabilitation*, 4, 46-54.

Dams-O'Connor, K., Tsaousides, T., Cantor, J., & Gordon, W.A. (in press). Integrating top-down and bottom-up interventions after traumatic brain injury: A Synergistic Approach to Neurorehabilitation. *Mount Sinai Journal of Medicine*.

Dahlberg, C.A., Cusick, C.P., Hawley, L.A. et.al. (2007) Treatment efficacy of social communication skills training after traumatic brain injury: A randomized treatment and deferred treatment controlled trial. *Archives of Physical Medicine and Rehabilitation*, 88, 1561-1573.

Dawson, D.R., Gaya, A., Hunt, A., Levine, B., Lemsky, C., & Polatajko, H.J. (2009) Using the Cognitive Orientation to Cognitive Performance (CO-OP) with adults with executive dysfunction following traumatic brain injury. *Canadian Journal of Occupational Therapy*, 76, 115-127.

Diller, L., & Weinberg, J. (1977) Hemi-inattention in rehabilitation: The evolution of a rational remediation program. *Advances in Neurology*, 18, 63-82.

Diller, L., Weinberg, J., Piasetsky, E., Ruckdeschel-Hibbard, M., Egelko, S., Scotzin, M., Couniotakis, J., & Gordon, W. (1980) *Methods for the evaluation and treatment of the visual perceptual difficulties of right brain damaged individuals*. Manual supplement to the 8th Annual Workshop for Rehabilitation Professionals. New York: Institute of Rehabilitation Medicine, New York University Medical Center.

Donaghy, S. & Williams, W. (1998) A new protocol for training severely impaired patients in usage of memory journals. *Brain Injury*, 12, 1061-1076.

Ehlhardt, L., Sohlberg, M., Glang, A. & Albin, R. (2005) TEACH-M: A pilot study evaluating an instructional sequence for persons with impaired memory and executive functions. *Brain Injury*, 19, 569-583.

Evans, J.J., Wilson, B.A., Schuri, U., Andrade, J., Baddeley, A., Bruna, O., et al.. (2000) A comparison of errorless and trial-and-error learning methods for teaching individuals with acquired memory deficits. *Neuropsychological Rehabilitation*, 10, 67-101.

Fasotti, L., Kovacs, F., Eling, P., & Brouwer, W. (2000) Time pressure management as a compensatory strategy training after closed head injury. *Neuropsychological Rehabilitation*, 10, 47-65.

Fish, J., Evans, J.J., Nimmo, M., Martin, E., Kersel, D., Bateman, A., Wilson, B.A., & Manly, T. (2006) Rehabilitation of executive dysfunction following brain injury: "Content-free" cueing improves everyday prospective memory performance. *Neuropsychologia 2006*, 44, 1318-1330.

Flanagan, S., McDonald, S., & Togher, L. (1995) Evaluation of the BRISS as a measure of social skills in the traumatically brain injured. *Brain Injury*, 9, 321-38.

Fleming, J. & Ownsworth, T. (2006) A review of awareness interventions in brain injury rehabilitation. *Neuropsychological Rehabilitation*, 16, 474-500.

Giacino, J. & Cicerone, K. (1998) Varieties of deficit unawareness after brain injury. *Journal of Head Trauma Rehabilitation*, 13, 1-15.

Glasgow, R. (1977) Case studies on remediating memory deficits in brain damaged individuals. *Journal of Clinical Psychology*, 33, 1049-1054.

Godefroy, O. & Rousseaux, M. (1997) Novel decision making in patients with prefrontal or posterior brain damage. *Neurology*, 49, 695-701.

Gordon, W.A., Hibbard, M.R., Egelko, S., Diller, L., Shaver, M.S., Lieberman, A., & Ragnarsson, K. (1985) Perceptual remediation in patients with right brain damage: A comprehensive program. *Archives of Physical Medicine and Rehabilitation*, 66, 353-359.

Gordon, W.A., Cantor, J., Ashman, T., & Brown, M. (2006) Treatment of Post-TBI Executive Dysfunction: Application of Theory to Clinical Practice. *Journal of Head Trauma Rehabilitation*, 21, 156–167.

Goverover, Y., Johnston, M., Toglia, J., & DeLuca, J. (2007) Treatment to improve self awareness in persons with acquired brain injury. *Brain Injury*, 21, 913-923.

Gray, J.M., Robertson, I., Pentland, B., & Anderson, S. (1992) Microcomputer-based attentional retraining after brain damage: A randomized group controlled trial. *Neuropsycholological Rehabilitation*, 2, 97-115.

Hawley, L. & Newman, J. (2008) *Group Interactive Structured Treatment – GIST: For Social Competence*. Denver, CO, 2006; updated 2008; (originally titled Social Skills and Traumatic Brain Injury: A Workbook for Group Treatment; and Social Problem-solving Group, 2003). www.braininjurysocialcompetence.com.

Hawley, L, & Newman, J. (2006) *Social skills and traumatic brain injury: a workbook for group treatment*. Authors. www.braininjurysocialcompetence.com.

Hawley, L., & Newman, J. (2010) Group Interactive Structured Treatment (GIST): A social competence intervention for individuals with brain injury. *Brain Injury*, 24:11, 1292-1297.

Kaschel, R., Della Sala, S., Cantagallo, A., Fahlbock, A., Laaksonen, R., & Kazen, M. (2002) Imagery mnemonics for the rehabilitation of memory: A randomized group controlled trial. *Neuropsychological Rehabilitation*, 12, 127-153.

Kay, T. & Cavallo, M.M. (1994) The family system: Impact, assessment, and intervention. In Silver, J.M., Yudofsky, S.C., & Hales, R.E. (Eds) *Neuropsychiatry of Traumatic Brain Injury*. Washington DC: American Psychiatric Press.

Kennedy, M.R.T., Coelho, C., Turkstra, L., Ylvisaker, M., Sohlberg, M.M., Yorkston, K., Chiou, H.H., & Kan, P.F. (2008) Intervention for executive functions after traumatic brain injury: A systematic review, meta-analysis and clinical recommendations. *Neuropsychological Rehabilitation*, 12: 3, 257-199.

Langenbahn, D., Rath, J., Hradil, A., Litke, D., Tucker, J. & Diller, L. (2008) Poster 8: A new approach to remediating problem-solving deficits in outpatients with moderate-to-severe cognitive impairments. *Archives of Physical Medicine and Rehabilitation*, 89, 1849-2040.

Lawson, M. & Rice, D. (1989) Effects of training in the use of executive strategies on a verbal memory problem resulting from closed head injury. *Journal of Clinical and Experimental Neuropsychology*, 11, 842-854.

Levine, B., Robertson, I. et al. (2000) Rehabilitation of executive function: An experimental-clinical validation of Goal Management Training, *Journal of the International Neuropsychological Society*, 6, 299-312.

McCarthy, M. et al. (2002) The role of imagery in the rehabilitation of neglect in severely disabled brain-injured adults. *Archives of Clinical Neuropsychology*, 17, 407-422.

McDonald, S., Tate, R., Togher, L. et al. (2008) Social skills treatment for people with severe, chronic acquired brain injuries: A multicenter trial. *Archives of Physical Medicine and Rehabilitation*, 89, 1648-1659.

Manly, T., Hawkins, K., Evans, J., Woldt, K. & Robertson, K.H. (2002) Rehabilitation of executive function: facilitation of effective goal management on complex tasks using periodic auditory alerts. *Neuropsychologia*, 40, 271-281.

Medd, J., & Tate, R. (2000) Evaluation of an anger management therapy programme following acquired brain injury: A preliminary study. *Neuropsychological Rehabilitation*, 10, 185-201.

Miechenbaum, D.H., & Goodman, J. (1971) Training impulsive children to talk to themselves: A means of developing self-control. *Journal of Abnormal Psychology*, 77, 115-126.

Miller, G.A., Galanter, E. & Pribram, K.H. (1960) Plans and the Structure of Behavior. New York: Holt, Rinehart and Winston, Inc.

Mirsky, A.F., Bruno, J.A, Duncan, C.C., Ahearn, M. & Sheppard, G.K. (1991) Analysis of the elements of attention: A neuropsychological approach. *Neuropsychology Review*, 2, 109-145.

Niemeier, J. (1998) The Lighthouse Strategy: Use of visual imagery technique to treat visual inattention in stroke patients. *Brain Injury*, 12, 399-406.

Niemeier, J.P., Cifu, D.X., & Kishore, R. (2001) The Lighthouse Strategy: Improving the functional status of patients with unilateral neglect after stroke and brain injury using a visual imagery intervention. *Top Stroke Rehabilitation*, 8:2, 10–18.

Ownsworth, T.L., & McFarland, K. (1999) Memory remediation in long-term acquired brain injury: two approaches in diary training. *Brain Injury*, 13:8, 605-626.

Ownsworth, T., McFarland, K. & Young, R. (2000) Self-awareness and psychosocial functioning following acquired brain injury: An evaluation of a group support programme. *Neuropsychological Rehabilitation*, 10, 465-484.

Pizzamiglio, L., Antonucci, G., Judica, A., Montenero, P., Razzano, C. & Zoccolotti, P. (1992) Cognitive rehabilitation of the hemineglect disorder in chronic patients with unilateral right brain damage. *Journal of Clinical and Experimental Neuropsychology*, 14, 901-923.

Rath, J., Simon, D., Langenbahn, D., Sherr, R., & Diller, L. (2003) Group treatment of problem-solving deficits in outpatients with traumatic brain injury: A randomized outcome study. *Neuropsychological Rehabilitation*, 13, 461-488.

Rizzolatti, R. & Camarda, R. (1987) Neural circuits for spatial attention and unilateral neglect. In Jeannerod, M. (Eds) *Neurophysiological and Neuropsychological Aspects of Spatial Neglect* (pp 289-313). Amsterdam: Elsevier.

Robertson, I. et al. (1998) Rehabilitation of unilateral neglect: Improving function by contralesional limb activation. *Neuropsychological Rehabilitation*, 8, 19-29.

Robertson, I. (1996) *Goal Management Training: A Clinical Manual*. Cambridge, U.K.: PsyConsult.

Robertson, I. & North, N. (1993) Active and passive activation of left limbs: Influence on visual and sensory neglect. *Neuropsychologia*, 31, 293-300.

Robinson, R.G. & Jorge, R. (1994) Mood Disorders. In Silver, J.M., Yudofsky, S.C., & Hales, R.E. (Eds) *Neuropsychiatry of Traumatic Brain Injury*. Washington DC: American Psychiatric Press.

Samuel, C. et al. (2000) Rehabilitation of very severe unilateral neglect by visuo-spatio-motor cueing: two single case studies. *Neuropsychological Rehabilitation*, 10, 385-399.

Schlund, M. (1999) Self awareness: effects of feedback and review on verbal self reports and remembering following brain injury. *Brain Injury*, 13, 375-380.

Sherr, R.L., Rath, J.F., Langenbahn, D.M., Litke, D.R., Hradil, A., Cascio, D.P., Yi, A., & Diller, L. (2008) Treatment for emotional self-regulation and problem-solving deficits in adults with moderate to severe cognitive deficits [abstract]. *Journal of the International Neuropsychological Society*, 14: S1, 239.

Shiffrin, R. & Schneider, W. (1977) Controlled and automatic human information processing: Perceptual learning, automatic attending and a general theory. *Psychological Review*, 84, 127-190.

Sohlberg, M. (2005) External aids for management of memory impairment. In High, W., Sander, A., Struchen, K.M. & Hart, K.A. (Eds) *Rehabilitation for Traumatic Brain Injury*. New York: Oxford University Press.

Sohlberg, M., Avery, J., Kennedy, M., Ylvisaker, M., Coelho, C., Turkstra, L. & Yorkston, K. (2003) Practice guidelines for direct attention training. *Journal of Medical Speech-Language Pathology*, 11, 19-39.

Sohlberg, M., Johnson, L., Paule, L., Raskin, S. & Mateer, C. (2001) Attention Process Training II: A program to address attentional deficits for persons with mild cognitive dysfunction. Puyallup, WA: Lash & Associates Publishing/Training Inc.

Sohlberg, M. & Mateer, C. (1987a) Effectiveness of an attention training programme. *Journal of Clinical and Experimental Neuropsychology*, 9, 117-130.

Sohlberg, M. & Mateer, C. (1987b) *Attention Process Training Assessment*. Puyallup, WA: Association for Neuropsychological Research and Development.

Sohlberg, M.A. & Mateer, C.A. (1989) *Introduction to Cognitive Rehabilitation Theory and Practice*. New York: Guilford Press.

Sohlberg, M. & Mateer, C. (2001) *Cognitive Rehabilitation: An Integrative Neuropsychological Approach.* New York: The Guilford Press.

Sohlberg, M., McLaughlin, K., Pavese, A., Heidrich, A. & Posner, M. (2000) Evaluation of attention process training and brain injury education in persons with acquired brain injury. *Journal of Clinical and Experimental Neuropsychology,* 22, 656-676.

Teuber, H.L. (1964) The riddle of frontal lobe function in man. In Warren, J.M. & Akert, K. (Eds) *The Frontal Granular cortex and Behavior* (pp 410-444). New York: McGraw-Hill.

Thickpenny-Davis, K.L., & Barker-Collow, S.L. (2007) Evaluation of a structured group format memory rehabilitation program for adults following brain injury. *Journal of Head Trauma Rehabilitation,* 22, 303-313.

Toglia, J., & Kirk, U. (2000) Understanding awareness deficits following brain injury. *NeuroRehabilitation,* 15, 57-70.

Von Cramon, D., Von Cramon, G., & Mai, N. (1991) Problem-solving deficits in brain-injured patients: A therapeutic approach. *Neuropsychological Rehabilitation,* 1, 45-64.

Webster, J.S., McFarland, P.T., Rapport, L.J., Morrill, B., Roades, L.A. & Abadee, P.S. (2001) Computer assisted training for improving wheelchair mobility in unilateral neglect patients. *Archives of Physical Medicine & Rehabilitation,* 82, 769-775.

Weinberg, J., Diller, L, Gordon, W.A., Gerstman, L.J., Lieberman, A., Lakin, P., Hodges, G., & Ezrachi, O. (1977) Visual scanning training effect on reading-related tasks in acquired right brain damage. *Archives of Physical Medicine and Rehabilitation,* 58, 479-486.

Weinberg, J., Diller, L., Gordon, W.A., Gerstman, L.J., Lieberman, A., Lakin, P., Hodges, G., & Ezrachi, O. (1979) Training sensory awareness and spatial organization in people with right brain damage. *Archives of Physical Medicine and Rehabilitation,* 60, 491-496.

West, R. (1995) Compensatory strategies for age-associated memory impairment. In Baddeley, A.D., Wilson, B.A. & Watts, F.N. (Eds), *Handbook of Memory Disorders* (pp 481-500). New York: Wiley.

Wiart, L., Bon Saint Come, A., Debelleix, X., Petit, H., Joseph, P.A., Mazaux, J.M. et al.. (1997) Unilateral neglect syndrome rehabilitation by truck rotation and scanning training. *Archives of Physical Medicine and Rehabilitation,* 78, 424-429.

Wilson, B. (2009) *Memory Rehabilitation: Integrating Theory and Practice.* New York: Guilford Press.

Wilson, B.A. (1987) *Rehabilitation of Memory.* New York: Guilford Press.

Wilson, F. et al. (2000) The effect of contralesional limb activation and sustained attention training for self-care programmes in unilateral spatial neglect. *Restorative Neurology and Neuroscience,* 16, 1-4.

Winkens, I., Van Heugten, C., Wade, D., & Fasotti, L. (2009) Training patients in Time Pressure Management: A cognitive strategy for mental slowness. *Clinical Rehabilitation,* 23, 79-90.

Winkens, I., Van Heugten, C., Fasotti, L., & Wade, D. (2009) Reliability and validity of two new instruments for measuring aspects of mental slowness in the daily lives of stroke patients. *Neuropsychological Rehabilitation,* 19, 64-85.

Wood, R. & McMillan, T. (2001) *Neurobehavioural Disability and Social Handicap Following Traumatic Brain Injury.* Philadelphia: Psychology Press.

Worthington, A. (1996) Cueing strategies in neglect dyslexia. *Neuropsychological Rehabilitation,* 6, 1-17.

Ylvisaker, M. & Feeney, T. (1998) *Collaborative Brain Injury Intervention: Positive Everyday Routines.* San Diego: Singular.

Zencius, A., Wesolowski, M.D., & Burke, W.H. (1990) A comparison for four memory strategies with traumatically brain-injured clients. *Brain Injury,* 4, 33-38.

Appendix A: Strategic and Tactical Goal Writing

A.1 Executive Dysfunction

BI-ISIG Cognitive Rehabilitation Task Force Recommendations

Practice Standard: Metacognitive strategy training for executive dysfunction and impairments of emotional self-regulation after TBI, and as a component of interventions for deficits in attention, neglect and memory. This includes self-monitoring and self-regulation

Practice Guideline: Training in formal problem-solving strategies and their application to everyday situations and functional activities during post-acute rehabilitation after TBI.

Practice Option: Group based interventions may be considered for remediation of executive and problem-solving deficits after TBI.

Goal Writing for the Treatment of Deficits in Executive Functioning

Strategic: Initial Monthly Goals/ Problem-Solving Protocol

- Initiate _____ (e.g., Acquisition, Application, Adaptation) stage of formal problem-solving protocol using the _____ (e.g., Goal-Plan-Do-Review, WSTC, etc.) method and implement as able.
- Initiate metacognitive strategy training to address _____.

Tactical: Follow-up/Specific Monthly Goals

- Patient will perform _____1_____ task, at _____2_____ level of difficulty, with _____3_____ accuracy/speed or _____4_____ assistance, using _____5_____ equipment/strategies/modifications.

(1) Types of Tasks

Impairment Level

- Divided attention tasks
- Problem-solving/reasoning tasks
- Sequencing tasks
- Organization tasks
- Planning tasks
- Flexibility tasks

Functional Level

- Functional clinic tasks requiring _____ ability
- Functional household tasks requiring _____ ability
- Functional community tasks requiring _____ ability
- Functional work-related tasks requiring _____ ability

(5) Types of Strategies

- Goal-Plan-Do-Review
- WSTC
- Self-talk

Examples

- Patient will perform simple problem-solving tasks with 80% accuracy.
- Patient will perform simple functional household tasks requiring planning ability with Min. Assistance.
- Patient will perform complex in-clinic tasks requiring problem-solving ability with Min. Assistance using Goal-Plan-Do-Review strategy.
- Patient will perform complex functional household tasks requiring organizational ability with 100% accuracy using Memory Notebook and WSTC strategies.

A.2 Memory Impairment

BI-ISIG Cognitive Rehabilitation Task Force Recommendations

Practice Standard: For those with mild impairment, the committee recommends the use of memory strategy training including the use of internalized strategies (e.g., visual imagery, mnemonics) and external memory compensations (e.g., notebooks, electronic devices).

Practice Guideline: For those with moderate to severe impairment, the committee recommends only the use of external compensations (including notebooks, electronic devices, etc.) with direct application to functional activities.

Practice Option: For people with severe memory impairments after TBI, errorless learning techniques may be effective for learning specific skills or knowledge, with limited transfer to novel tasks or reduction in overall functional memory problems.

Practice Option: Group based interventions may be considered for remediation of memory deficits after TBI.

Goal Writing for Deficits in Memory

Strategic/General Monthly Goals: Memory Book Protocol
- Initiate/complete acquisition stage of memory book protocol.
- Initiate/complete application stage of memory book protocol.
- Initiate/complete adaptation stage of memory book protocol.
- Implement modified memory book protocol, _____ stage.

Strategic: Memory Strategy Training
- Initiate internalized/memory strategy training including visual imagery and self-talk procedures.

Tactical: Follow-up/Specific Monthly Goals
- Patient will recall/perform_____ 1_____ , at _____ 2_____ level of difficulty, with _____3_____ accuracy or _____4_____cues/assistance, using_____5_____equipment/strategies/modifications.

(1) Types of Tasks
Impairment Level
- List learning tasks
- Story memory tasks
- Prospective memory tasks
- Visuospatial memory tasks
- Etc.

Functional Level
- Functional clinic tasks requiring _____ ability
- Functional household tasks requiring _____ ability
- Functional community tasks requiring _____ ability
- Functional work-related tasks requiring _____ ability
- Others

(5) Types of Strategies
- Internal strategies/Mnemonics
- Memory Notebook
- Electronic device

Examples
- Patient will recall simple autobiographical information with 80% accuracy using Memory Notebook.
- Patient will learn and recall names with 70% accuracy using internal strategies.
- Patient will perform complex functional in-clinic tasks requiring prospective memory with 70% accuracy using Memory Notebook.
- Patient will perform simple household tasks requiring list learning with minimal assistance using Memory Notebook strategy.

A.3 Attention Impairment

BI-ISIG Cognitive Rehabilitation Task Force Recommendations

Practice Standard: Remediation of attention is recommended during post-acute rehabilitation after TBI. Remediation of attention deficits after TBI should include direct attention training and metacognitive training to promote development of compensatory strategies and foster generalization to real world tasks. Insufficient evidence exists to distinguish the effects of specific attention training during acute recovery and rehabilitation from spontaneous recovery, or from more general cognitive interventions.

Practice Option: Computer-based interventions may be considered as an adjunct to clinician-guided treatment for the remediation of attention deficits after TBI or stroke. Sole reliance on repeated exposure and practice on computer-based tasks without some involvement and intervention by a therapist is NOT recommended.

Goal Writing for Deficits in Attention and Concentration

Strategic Monthly Goals: APT Protocol
- Initiate Strategy Training to address impairment in _____ (sustained, alternating, selective, divided attention).
- Initiate APT Protocol to address _____.
- Initiate Time Pressure Management to address _____.
- Consider psychostimulant or other medication to enhance attention/concentration.

Tactical: APT Goals

Sustained Attention
- Simple sustained attention tasks with _____ accuracy/speed and _____ cues
- Moderate sustained attention tasks with _____ accuracy/speed and _____ cues
- Complex sustained attention tasks with _____ accuracy/speed and _____ cues

Alternating Attention
- Simple alternating attention tasks with _____ accuracy/speed and _____ cues
- Moderate alternating attention tasks with _____ accuracy/speed and _____ cues
- Complex alternating attention tasks with _____ accuracy/speed and _____ cues

Selective Attention
- Simple selective attention tasks with _____ accuracy/speed and _____ cues
- Moderate selective attention tasks with _____ accuracy/speed and _____ cues
- Complex selective attention tasks with _____ accuracy/speed and _____ cues

Divided Attention
- Simple divided attention tasks with _____ accuracy/speed and _____ cues
- Moderate divided attention tasks with _____ accuracy/speed and _____ cues
- Complex divided attention tasks with _____ accuracy/speed and _____ cues

Tactical: Follow-up/Specific Monthly Goals
- Patient will perform _____1_____ at _____2_____ level of difficulty, with _____3_____ accuracy/speed or _____4_____ cues/assistance, using _____5_____ equipment/strategies/modifications.

(1) Type of Tasks
Impairment Level
- Sustained attention task
- Alternating attention task
- Selective attention task
- Divided attention task

Functional Tasks

- Functional household tasks requiring _____ ability
- Functional community tasks requiring _____ ability
- Functional work-related tasks requiring _____ ability
- Others

Examples

- Patient will perform simple selective attention tasks with 80% accuracy.
- Patient will reduce time to completion on tasks of complex sustained attention by 20%.
- Patient will perform simple functional household tasks requiring sustained attention with minimal assistance.
- Patient will perform complex in-clinic tasks requiring alternating attention with minimal assistance.
- Patient will perform complex functional household tasks requiring divided attention with 100% accuracy.

A.4 Visuospatial Strategies

BI-ISIG Cognitive Rehabilitation Task Force Recommendations

Practice Standard: Visuospatial rehabilitation that includes visual scanning training is recommended for left visual neglect after right hemisphere stroke.

Practice Guideline: The use of isolated microcomputer exercises to treat left neglect after stroke does not appear effective and is NOT recommended.

Practice Option: Limb activation or electronic technologies for visual scanning training in those with neglect. It also suggested that systematic training of visuospatial and organizational skills may be considered for those with right cerebral hemisphere dysfunction causing visual perceptual deficits without visual neglect, but not for those with a left hemisphere stroke or TBI. It also considers the possibility that computer-based interventions may be helpful in extending damaged visual fields in those with stroke or TBI.

Goal-Writing for Treatment of Visual Neglect

Strategic: Protocol for Neglect

- Initiate protocol for visual neglect, including limb activation strategies and scanning strategies (if appropriate).

Tactical: Follow-up/Specific Monthly Goals

- Patient will perform _____1_____, at _____2_____ level of difficulty, with _____3_____ accuracy/speed or _____4_____ assistance, using _____5_____ equipment/strategies/modifications.

(1) Type of tasks

Impairment Level

- Visual scanning tasks
- Visuospatial construction tasks
- Visuospatial perception tasks

Functional Level

- Functional clinic tasks requiring _____ ability
- Functional household tasks requiring _____ ability
- Functional community tasks requiring _____ ability
- Functional work-related tasks requiring _____ ability

(5) Type of Strategies

- Visual scanning
- Limb activation strategies

Examples

- Patient will perform simple visual scanning tasks with 80% accuracy.
- Patient will perform complex functional household tasks requiring scanning ability with minimal assistance, using Lighthouse strategy.
- Patient will perform complex in-clinic tasks requiring scanning ability with Min. Assistance using limb activation strategy.
- Patient will perform complex functional household tasks requiring organizational ability with 100% accuracy using combined strategies of limb activation and scanning.

A.5 Sample Template of Monthly Goals

Month 1:   Strategic Goals

1. Begin Acquisition stage of Memory Notebook training.
2. Begin Acquisition stage of problem-solving protocol, if able.

Tactical Goals

1. Patient will perform simple problem-solving tasks with 80% accuracy.
2. Patient will perform simple functional household tasks requiring planning ability.
3. Patient will recall simple autobiographical information with 80% accuracy using Memory Notebook.
4. Patient will learn and recall names with 70% accuracy using internal strategies.

Month 2:   Strategic Goals

1. Begin Application stage of Memory Notebook training, if able.
2. Begin/Continue with Acquisition stage of problem-solving, if able.
3. Begin self instructional strategy, if able.

Tactical Goals

1. Patient will perform complex in-clinic tasks requiring problem-solving ability with minimal assistance using Goal-Plan-Do-Review strategy.
2. Patient will perform complex functional household tasks requiring organizational ability with 100% accuracy using Memory Notebook and WSTC strategies.
3. Patient will perform complex functional in-clinic tasks requiring prospective memory with 70% accuracy using Memory Notebook.
4. Patient will perform simple household tasks requiring list learning with minimal assistance using Memory Notebook strategy.

Appendix B: General/Non-Specific Forms

B.1 Acquisition Record

APPLICATION RECORD: Multiple Tasks

Name: _____

Dates: _____

DATES and TRIALS

TASKS									
1									
2									
3									
4									
5									
6									
7									
8									
Comments									
Staff initials									

Outcome:

+ = Accurate and complete

– = Inaccurate or incomplete

KEY: Level of Cueing:

I = Spontaneous / Independent

Min = Verbal Cues (e.g. you will want to remember this…)

Max = "Write this down"

DIRECTIONS: Each staff will indicate the level of cueing needed for each trial along with the outcome. Staff can add comments if needed and initial their observation.

B.2 Acquisition Record: Multiple Tasks

ADAPTATION RECORD: Multiple Tasks

Name: _____

DATES and TRIALS

DATE	TASK	LEVEL OF CUEING NEEDED	OUTCOME /COMMENTS

KEY: **Level of Cueing:**

I = Spontaneous / Independent

Min = Verbal Cues (e.g. you will want to remember this...)

Max = "Write this down"

Outcome:

+ = Accurate and complete

– = Inaccurate and incomplete

DIRECTIONS: Each staff will indicate the level of cueing needed for each trial along with the outcome. Staff can add comments if needed and initial their observation.

B.3 Adaptation Record: Multiple Tasks, Alternate Form

ADAPTATION RECORD: Multiple Tasks

Name: _____

DATES and TRIALS

TASKS									
1									
2									
3									
4									
5									
6									
7									
8									

KEY: Level of Cueing:

I = Spontaneous / Independent

Min = Verbal Cues (e.g. you will want to remember this...)

Max = Write this down

Outcome:

+ = Accurate and complete

− = Inaccurate or incomplete

DIRECTIONS: Each staff will indicate the level of cueing needed for each trial along with the outcome.

FIRST EDITION

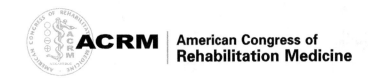

ACRM | American Congress of
Rehabilitation Medicine

The American Congress of Rehabilitation Medicine (ACRM) is an organization of rehabilitation professionals dedicated to serving people with disabling conditions by supporting research that:

- promotes health, independence, productivity, and quality of life,
- meets the needs of rehabilitation clinicians and people with disabilities.

In order to enhance current and future research and knowledge translation, ACRM:

- assists researchers in improving their investigations and dissemination of findings
- educates providers to deliver best practices, and
- advocates for funding of future rehabilitation research.

The ACRM is a global community of both researchers and consumers of research, in the field of rehabilitation. ACRM is the only professional association representing all members of the multidisciplinary rehabilitation team, including: physicians, psychologists, rehabilitation nurses, occupational therapists, physical therapists, speech therapists, recreation specialists, case managers, rehabilitation counselors, vocational counselors, and disability management specialists.

ACRM is dedicated to:

- serving as an advocate for public policy and legislative issues that support individuals with disabilities and providers of rehabilitation services,

- helping develop innovative and cost-effective models of collaborative care and comprehensive rehabilitation management,

- leading research efforts that examine and develop the most effective clinical technology and treatment paradigms, and

- initiating dialogue with payers and regulators to communicate the collaborative care models that produce positive rehabilitation outcomes.

MISSION

ACRM enhances the lives of people living with disabilities through a multidisciplinary approach to rehabilitation. As leaders in the physical medicine and rehabilitation field, ACRM promotes innovative research, new technologies, sharing information, and encourages evidence-based practices in clinical settings.

LEADERSHIP ROLE

As rehabilitation science continues to evolve, ACRM's goal is to keep the community connected by creating opportunities to exchange and share information among clinical practitioners, rehabilitation researchers, knowledge brokers, research funders, provider organizations, healthcare payers, and industry regulators.

The ACRM encourages leaders in rehabilitation to identify current best practices and best providers at all levels of care, and share this information via education meetings and the journal, *Archives of Physical Medicine and Rehabilitation*.

The ACRM aims to support multidisciplinary leadership and practice innovation to ensure that people living with chronic disease or disability have access to effective rehabilitation services throughout their lives.

The ACRM serves as a forum for creating and discussing new treatment paradigms that take into account the composition of the rehabilitation team, the duration of care, and the venues required to achieve optimal functional outcomes for people with chronic disease and disabilities.

www.ACRM.org

MEMBERSHIP APPLICATION

www.ACRM.org

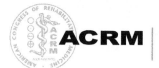 **ACRM** | American Congress of **Rehabilitation Medicine**

O Dr.   O Ms.   O Mr.   Referred by _____

First Name_____ Last Name_____ Credentials _____

PERSONAL

I prefer to receive O email O mail at this address.

Home Address _____

_____

City _____St/Province _____

Zip _____ Country _____

Tel _____ Mobile_____

Email_____

MEMBERSHIP CATEGORIES & DUES (USD) *choose one*

O **Regular**   **$350**
   BA/BS in medical rehabilitation or related field
   actively engaged in the practice, administration,
   education or research of medical rehabilitation.

O **International**   **$350**
   Resides outside the US and qualifies for Regular.

O **Consumer**   **$350**
   For people with disabilities and caregivers who use
   rehabilitation services and/or research.

O **Early Career**   **$150**
   For professionals during the first 2 years after
   completion of post-graduate studies.

   Completion Date (mo/yr) _____

O **Resident, Student or Fellow**   **$ 85**
   Enrolled in an accredited school of medicine or
   approved graduate or undergraduate program or
   fellowship in a medical rehabilitation discipline.

   Graduation Date (mo/year) _____

   Training Director (name, credentials and email)

   _____

   _____

   _____

SPECIAL INTEREST & NETWORKING GROUPS

Membership includes affiliation with **all** ACRM community
forums. Please select all community forums in which you
wish to participate.

O Brain Injury Interdisciplinary (BI-ISIG)
O Outcome Measurement Networking Group (OMNG)
O Spinal Cord Injury (SCI-SIG)
O Stroke Networking Group (SNG)

Membership Dues $_____

Donations (unspecified) $_____

Wilkerson Fund Donation $_____

Total $_____

BUSINESS

I prefer to receive O email O mail at this address.

Organization _____

Title _____

Department _____

Employer Address _____

_____

_____

City _____St/Province _____

Zip _____Country _____

Tel _____Mobile _____

Email_____

SPECIALIZATIONS *check all that apply*

O Bioengineering   O Psychology
O Biostatistics / Clinical   O Physiatry
   Research   O Physical Therapy
O Case Manager   O Psychiatry
O Clinical Epidemiology   O Recreation Therapy
O Counseling, Pastoral   O Rehabilitation Nursing
O Counseling,   O Rehabilitation
   Rehabilitation   Psychology
O Counseling, Vocational   O Social Work
O Dietetics I Nutrition   O Speech I Language
O Neurology I   Pathology
   Neurosurgery   O Other Physician
O Neuropsychology
O Occupational Therapy   _____
O Pediatrics
                               O Other_____

Work Function *choose one*

O Administrator   O Program Evaluator
O Clinician   O Researcher
O Consultant   O Student
O Educator   O Other_____
O Payer

Payment Options Payment accepted in U.S. dollars only.

Check payable to ACRM
Mail to: PO Box 759272, Baltimore, MD 21275-9272

Credit Card
Fax to: +1.866.692.1619
Email to: MemberServices@ACRM.org

O VISA   O MasterCard   O Amex   O Discover

Card #_____ Exp_____

Signature _____

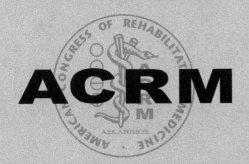

TREMENDOUS MEMBER VALUE
MONETARY & IMMEASURABLES

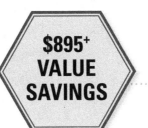
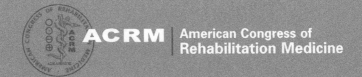

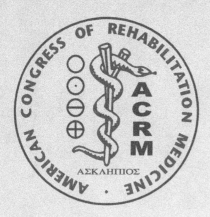

THANK YOU ACRM INSTITUTIONAL MEMBERS

PLATINUM LEVEL
Rusk Institute of Rehabilitation Medicine

GOLD LEVEL
Shepherd Center
Spaulding Rehabilitation Network

SILVER LEVEL
Craig Hospital
Pate Rehabilitation Endeavors, Inc
Rehabilitation Hospital of Indiana
TIRR Memorial Hermann

BRONZE LEVEL
Courage Center
Ohio State University

Your decision to become an Institutional Member of ACRM demonstrates to the world your support of evidence-based innovation in rehabilitation.

Together we can significantly enhance the lives of people living with disabilities. Your support makes a positive impact in immeasurable ways. *Thank you!*

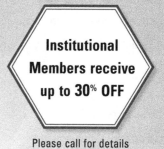

Institutional Members receive up to 30% OFF

Please call for details

ACRM | INSTITUTIONAL MEMBERSHIP INQUIRIES: | **JENNY RICHARD**
ACRM Director Member Services
EMAIL: jrichard@acrm.org
TEL: +1.703.574.5845

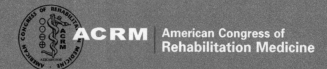

ACRM | American Congress of **Rehabilitation Medicine**

GLOBAL MULTIDISCIPLINARY REHABILITATION RESEARCH   TEL: +1.317.471.8760   www.ACRM.org

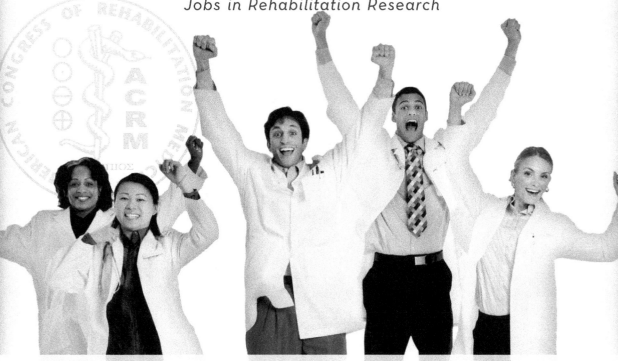
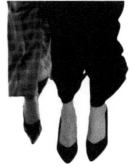
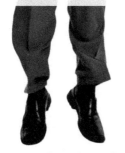
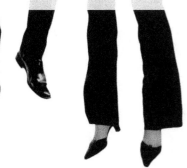
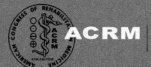

CPSIA information can be obtained
at www.ICGtesting.com
Printed in the USA
BVHW011116260820
587343BV00013B/379

9 780615 538877